Bus

STO

ACPL

DISCARDED

YO-ABQ-055

Living With Pain

DEC 19 '77

Barbara Wolf

LIVING
WITH
PAIN

Foreword by
JAMES G. WEPSIC, M.D

.

A Continuum Book
THE SEABURY PRESS · NEW YORK

The Seabury Press
815 Second Avenue · New York, New York 10017

Copyright © 1977 by Barbara B. Wolf. All rights reserved.
No part of this book may be reproduced, stored in a retrieval
system, or transmitted, in any form or by any means,
electronic, mechanical, photocopying, recording, or otherwise,
without the written permission of The Seabury Press.

Printed in the United States of America

Library of Congress Cataloging in Publication Data

Wolf, Barbara B.   Living with Pain.
(A Continuum book)   Bibliography:
1. Pain.   I. Title.
QP401.W64   616'.047   77–12194
ISBN 0–8164–9328–6

This book is affectionately
and gratefully dedicated to
ALAN M. ELKINS, M. D.

1983409

Contents

Foreword

Barbara Wolf has produced an excellent guide to feelings, responses, and effective social adaptation to persistent or "chronic" pain. Using her direct personal observations, candid introspection, exhaustive study, and a desire to make this work useful to other human beings, she has thoughtfully approached a subject which has not been treated in depth before. Recalling her own battle as a chain of reactions to an incapacitating series of nerve injuries, which left her unable to use her hands, she attempts to spare us from going down blind alleys she has visited and depicts the energy-draining short-term "easy outs." The armaments are personal hard thinking, discipline, and self-esteem. These essentials for grappling with pain are described in terms of their value in finding a workable solution both for persons with pain and the people they live with.

In my experience, this is a unique book. It provides a pragmatic approach to a personal crisis. This is a difficult task, for no two people have the same pain, the same social pressures, the same set of life experiences to draw on. Yet it is a task that has been well done. The vagaries, myths, and complex reactions that are bound together in pain are humanly dissected, not with a cold blade, but with wit and understanding. The result is comprehensible and useful to the person who has persistent pain, who fears it, or who faces it in a friend or family member. It is not a text of neurophysiology or psychology, nor does it pretend to be one. The reader is directed to those authorities if he wishes, but he should not overlook the value of this book, which lies in the treatment of what often seems to be an illogical situation in a rational way.

This book should be required reading for people concerned with pain.

James G. Wepsic, M. D.
Neurosurgeon,
Massachusetts General Hospital

Acknowledgments

Two distinct kinds of acknowledgment ought properly to be noted. Without the dedicated help and concern of many doctors and therapists I would never have been physically able to write this book. The hours they spent in treating me, in encouraging, teaching, and explaining were beyond price, and I thank them all. Fellow sufferers and friends gave me courage.

Special thanks to: James G. Wepsic, M. D., and Alan M. Elkins, M. D., who made it possible for me to gain access to medical libraries not ordinarily open to the public, who read the manuscript as it was written, and who offered valuable suggestions and comments; to my psychotherapist, Mrs. Betty G. Lockwood, who helped me to understand what I was undergoing; and to Frances M. Dyro, M.D. for information about acupuncture.

Not all the pain persons I interviewed wished to be identified; but I wish to thank Mr. Floyd Frisbee for his taped remarks and S. Z. for a chance to read some illuminating poems. Stephen Soreff, M.D., was kind enough to submit to an interview. And Priscilla and Don Webster were generous with reading proof and drawing diagrams.

My family helped beyond measure: my sister, Katherine B. Nuckolls, Ph. D., endured my questions and directed me toward answers; my daughters Julie and Jane gave generously of their ideas and imaginations; and my husband—who has had to suffer the sufferer—has been unfailingly encouraging and supportive.

Prologue

One day in January, 1973, six months after my first surgery, I found myself day-dreaming about those uncommon human beings who, for physical or psychological reasons, do not suffer pain—or do not react to pain as most of us do. Medical research has not yet developed a single explanation for this curious "abnormality." But my speculations had nothing to do with medical research or with single causes. It simply seemed to me, at the time, that I would have given anything, especially and specifically the right hand that was putting me through hell, for access to that happy state of no-pain. It made no difference at all that, rationally, I knew better than to make such a trade, even were it possible: Pain is, among other things, a signal that something is amiss in the body or in the mind or in both. To be incapable of feeling or responding to pain is to be without one of the more important defense mechanisms with which our bodies are equipped. It's the pain reflex that forces us to yank the finger away from a hot stove, for example. Without signals like pain

—fever is another—both patient and doctor are hampered in determining what an injury or disease is.

However, such fine rational considerations, such obvious common sense, had nothing to do with my day-dreaming. My right hand felt as if it were on fire. Sometimes the burning sensation was faint; sometimes it peaked to a level that I could only relate to barbecuing, or to what my imagination conceived a hamburger on a grill might feel, if it could. More than anything else, then, I wanted to break the contract between my neurological system and me. It was as if some malevolent stranger had intruded on my body, on my personal territory. Like an insomniac hearing footsteps downstairs, I could not find satisfaction in "realistic explanations." I knew better.

What I experienced in idle envy indicated, and still does, that rationality offers very little help to what I shall call the "pain person." To be sure, when one's mind is totally and fully engaged in some kind of exercise, the perception of pain is diminished, a fact with some far-reaching consequences. The pain I was experiencing that January had been magnified because I had necessarily taken a disability leave from my job. Hence I was denied the relief I had enjoyed during the fall of 1972 when I taught full time. That relief was, at best, transitory, but I welcomed it, without realizing why or how it worked. Fifty minutes' worth of the sound of my own and my students' voices provided fifty minutes of—well, not exactly no pain, but certainly *less* pain. I can distinctly remember lunches in the faculty dining room during which the same phenomenon recurred. Gossip, talk of salaries, news of administrative blunders, laughter—these caught me up, drew my attention away from the burning hand, gave me respite for a while.

But I found no respite at all in asking such questions as:

What is causing this? How long will it last? Will the scar tissue eventually go away? I did ask those questions, of course. Over and over again. The fact that I kept asking them, and kept being given the same answers, should have alerted me to the foolishness of trying to find reasons that my mind could not give me. I had been given physiological analyses of my problem. For instance, I learned that there is more than one kind of nerve fiber in the median nerve (I had never heard of the median nerve until it proclaimed its existence in late December, 1971). Some of those fibers in the nerve transmit sensation, some transmit pain, and others work muscles. Interesting, but a fact, not a means toward my personal goal—the cessation of burning.

For example, knowing what was going on in my hand did not stop what I later learned to call "fasciculation," a condition in which the muscles at the base of my thumb visibly jumped, spasmodically and painfully. Adding a new word to my vocabulary of medical terminology had some mild intellectual interest. But explaining a Shakespeare play or the nature of a complex-compound sentence was much more helpful; it enabled me to endure fasciculation as if it were going on in somebody else's thumb—at least most of the time.

During that January, however, I had nothing to force my attention away from my hand. Day-time television did not afford me the kind of compelling absorption necessary; nor did reading, except for some rare and gratefully devoured exceptions. Parties helped, although I wonder now whether the few I dared go to were as brilliant as I thought they were, and whether I was as scintillating a guest as I thought I was. (Did people comment on the way I hectically chattered and told jokes?) Sometimes I wallowed in self-pity, a disastrous wallow, since self-pity focuses attention on the pain and thereby intensifies it. Sometimes I curled up on the bed and cried helplessly, another disastrous activity for a pain person. And, like a surprising number of pain persons, I drank bourbon and gulped aspirin, the bourbon, at least, acting as a temporary method for achieving the I-don't-care effect, while doing its own dirty work. Again, *not* the recommended analgesic for someone in chronic pain.

And I felt guilty. Many pain persons do, since they are forever pestering their doctors for good news, and their families for sympathy and attention. Pain persons may feel themselves to be beggars, and only professional beggars escape the sense of guilt that attends us amateurs. In my case, the sense of guilt spread like smog over my relationships with other people. Friends wanted to help, offering to drive me to the market or to the movies. I regularly rebuffed them. "Now you *will* call me if you need a ride, won't you?" "Oh, certainly!" But I rarely did. It was as if the intruder, pain, had a gun at my head. I was a captive, struggling to be free, yet needing somehow to retain whatever rags of independent dignity I had left. Naturally, after a while, people stopped offering help. Everyone lost. I had my selfhood, but I had it all by myself. And my hand still burned.

A brief trip to England served as a break in what had become an almost precipitous spiral down into severe depression. Psychiatric help, both before and after the trip, aided in slowing the tailspin, as I began to learn about the emotional dimensions of my pain reactions.

A second surgical procedure in Boston afforded me not only three weeks of total remission, but three weeks of what bordered on giddiness: I was light-headed as well as light-hearted. On the trip back from Boston, my husband and I stopped for lunch at what was really a mediocre restaurant.

That the food was over-described, over-priced, and over-cooked mattered nothing at all to me. My hand had stopped hurting. One of the best hand surgeons in the country had removed what his assistant described as "about an inch and a half of scar tissue—hard as cement." The operation itself was in some ways a horror story (difficulties with regard to anesthesia), but it proved valuable in ways having little to do with my hand. It forced me to examine, with my psychotherapist, my childhood-born terror of doctors, pain, and hospitals. Consequently, later, potentially more frightening encounters with surgery were easier to face.

Physical relief and light-heartedness lasted only three weeks. Without warning, the intruder, pain, announced itself again. Its reappearance came as such a shock that I began thinking of my car in the garage, and of the merits of carbon monoxide. Self-destruction would destroy the intruder permanently. Permanent relief. Yet my emotional ties to my family and to life emerged as more powerful than I would have thought possible. Furthermore, although I know this in retrospect better than I did at the time, somewhere in the back of my mind began to stir a dim impulse or feeling that I wanted to fight back at, rather than succumb to, whatever it was that was invading my body.

In June, the hand surgeon, backing away from me as if I had a contagious disease, said he could under no circumstances operate again, even though his examination showed that the scar tissue had quickly and inexorably rebuilt itself. I quite understood his position. No surgeon wishes to undertake a procedure that is probably doomed to failure, unless the patient's life is at stake. In one sense, my life *was* at stake, but I could scarcely blame him. He did say that he thought there might be some help for the pain. He referred me to a neurosurgeon who, he said, specialized in a gadget that could turn pain off, even if it couldn't restore my hand to normal function.

The neurosurgeon's calm good sense, compassion, and wit carried me a little way into hope. For the first time, medical jargon and rational explanations began to make sense. They made sense because they were set in a context of hope and spoken by a surgeon who adopted me as a pain person, lonely and very frightened. The yellow brick road, with all its monstrous obstacles, had finally come to an end at the Emerald City.

The "gadget," called a neurostimulator, was implanted in July, 1973 (Senator Ervin's committee interviewed Haldeman and Ehrlichman or a television set at the foot of my bed in the hospital). When I was finally allowed to turn the "gadget" on, to learn to regulate and understand it (it requires a nine-volt transistor battery once every week to ten days), the intruder had been curbed. While the sensation created by the neurostimulator took some getting used to, it was certainly a vast improvement over the burning one. Pain no longer dominated my existence (although the search for fresh batteries now sometimes does). True, my right thumb did not function correctly, and still does not. But the pain had been controlled.

Well, even the Great Oz was not exactly all-powerful.

Because I am right-handed I had been busily engaged for several months in what I regarded as a remarkably successful crash course designed to convert myself into a southpaw. Kindergarten exercises: I drew big circles, printed with crayons on wide-ruled paper. I invigorated myself by taking large doses of inspirational stories about the handicapped who have learned to do the impossible with the improbable. During my last semester of full-time teaching I was able to write marginal notes in my Shakespeare text with my left hand. (That text, incidentally, looks like an archeological dig within which previous cultures have been carefully preserved. Pre-pain writing, left-handed writing, and post-neurostimulator writing. A short history of a pain person.)

Someone might have warned me, or I might have had more sense. The rigorous effort—and it was rigorous—to impose on my left hand what it could not take in the time I was giving it, created a strain that went on for months of correcting papers, preparing classes, cooking, driving a car (with an illegal "suicide knob"), coping with existence and bags of groceries. My best intentions exacted an ironic penalty. The same problem which had attacked my right hand suddenly attacked my left. The same old intruder, complete with the same old horrors, scared me back into the nightmare. So it was back to Boston and the hand surgeon. Surgery on my left hand. Initial relief. And this time, after only *two* weeks, pain again. To what extent my previous experiences speeded up the scar tissue growth after the surgery on my left hand (it was now January, 1974), I do not know precisely. Quite clearly, I was frightened of the possibility of a repeat performance. Also clear is psychiatric evidence that a patient's emotional condition can bring about astounding physical effects, including pain.

Then, in May, 1974, another "gadget," this one for my left hand. At last, after a summer's worth of physical and occupational therapy, interrupted for another operation to correct a problem with the implant (the House Judiciary Committee deliberating impeachment at the foot of the same bed in the same hospital), I was back at work, shaky, uncertain of myself, hampered by the constant need to evaluate the demands of a partial handicap.

It is axiomatic that no one wants to listen to the story of anyone else's pain, perhaps because we all have our own stories and would greatly prefer to be on the giving rather than the receiving end of such narratives. Indeed, in recent months I have avoided talking about my own experience; not only is the story too long, it is repetitive and therefore boring. So in writing this prologue I have deliberately omitted reference to the first operation on my right hand, and to the technical difficulties surrounding the initial diagnosis, and to the insensitivity displayed by a few doctors, and to the frustrations endured in getting from one specialist to another. In fact, I haven't even mentioned the official name for my disorder.

But one of the more hideous aspects of pain is that it isolates its victims, whether it attacks the emotions or the body. The pain person's cry includes the line "Nobody knows the trouble I've seen," because nobody on the outside of the invisible barricade can know precisely what it's like on the inside. All pain persons know what power loneliness possesses. When the intruder has us cowering and mute, we feel besieged; to make matters worse, we cannot find the means to break out.

Yet somehow the barricade must be breached, the voice must be found. A protracted siege, internalized and inexplicable, with the intruder constantly thwarting our attempts to preserve our own small peace of mind, is not fun. Attack is the best defense. Now that my intruder has been largely disarmed, I wish to give chase, to take the offensive, to put pain where it belongs. If I can do so, then perhaps some other pain person can do the same. How do we attack?

First, we have to define the intruder, give it a proper name. As the Israelites knew, getting hold of the proper name gives power over that which is otherwise shrouded in mystery. (They devised many substitutes for the name of God, but they kept his revealed name cryptic: JHVH. English translators of the Old Testament added vowels to give us "Jehovah.") Once we have identified the culprit, we can adopt a method of procedure. And since we are "attacking," the best method of procedure can be borrowed from experts on war. One of the best authorities is General Karl von Clausewitz, whose treatise *On War* remains a standard military textbook:

We must determine our *situation,* come to some understanding of our *problem,* outline a *strategy* to follow, and finally settle on the *tactics* that will best bring about a satisfactory conclusion to the siege.

In war, it is folly to react to a sticky *situation* by hasty resort to *tactical* solutions. The correct term for such a reaction is "panic." A panicky infantryman might retreat straight into an ambush; worse still, he might mistake friends for enemies. A panicky pain person might do much the same thing, might demand surgery or drugs without knowing how perilous the tactics of pain relief can be. In any event, without an adequate sense of what war is, both the infantryman and the pain person will be underequipped for what they must endure:

> As the human eye in a dark room dilates its pupil, draws in the little light that there is, partially distinguishes objects by degrees, and at last knows them quite well, so it is in War with the experienced soldier, whilst the novice is only met by pitch black night.
> —*von Clausewitz*

1

Definitions, or Name-Calling

The task of defining pain has cost a great many people a great deal of effort in what sometimes seems a less than successful endeavor. Some definitions are more entertaining than others. "An unpleasant sensation" seems scarcely adequate, although the phrase allows for a wide range of experiences and therefore includes everything from a persecution complex to a hangnail, including the mosquito bite. "A noxious stimulus" may seem more accurate, if one does not succumb, as I did, to musings about "noxious" substances, meaning poisons. Poisons have little to do with most pain, although the word "noxious" keeps creeping into medical literature having to do with the origins and treatments of pain. And "stimulus" is a little misleading, if only because pain involves more than "stimuli."

Stedman's Medical Dictionary gives us "Suffering, either physical or mental; an impression on the sensory nerves causing distress, or when extreme, agony. . . ." The use of "suffering" seems to me redundant, as does the frequently

11

used term "pain patient." ("Pain" means "suffering." "Patient" means "sufferer.") However, "either physical or mental" is decidedly well chosen. As we shall see, pain, as an intrusive force, includes far more than a simple neurological transaction. Emotional pain can cause physical pain; physical pain of long duration certainly causes emotional distress. But "impression on the sensory nerves" leads us to some rather unproductive hopes for relief, since not every form of pain can be diagnosed in terms having to do with the cells which make up our nervous systems.

But *Stedman's* goes one helpful step further: "The following self-explanatory terms . . . are used to describe p.: boring, burning, darting, shooting, piercing, lightning, nocturnal, jumping, crushing, tearing, lancinating, lacerating, grinding, throbbing, acute, sharp, dull, aching. . . ."

Now we find ourselves moving away from the constricting limits of definition to the broader areas of adjectives and metaphors. Why this transition is fruitful has much to do with our personal past histories. As children we probably experienced the acute pain of a splinter. A splinter-intrusion has a certain quality or quantity about it that will later, in other circumstances, be described as "shooting." A splinter doesn't "crush," it doesn't "grind" or "tear." Perhaps it throbs, but it does not occur only at night. Out of our own histories, we forge a vocabulary with which to deal with the intruder.* In effect, we create a highly developed language, one which doctors must learn to translate and even to speak fluently.

---

*Melzack and Torgerso have compiled a fascinating table of terms used to describe pain. Their table includes far more words than *Stedman's*. What is of interest is the fact that the terms can be classified as to emotional connotations. "Unbearable," for instance, has overtones of a moral or ethical nature. "On the Language of Pain," *Anaesthesiology,* Vol. 34, 1971, p. 50.

The adjectives and metaphors are necessary, simply because the unqualified statement "It hurts!" is of very little use to those who are trying to help. Two interns made up an illustrative dialogue for me:

"Oh, doctor, it hurts!"
"Where does it hurt?"
"Oh, gee, I don't know—*here!*" (pointing to chest)
"Can you tell me what kind of pain it is?"
"Oh, it just *hurts!*"
"Is it a crushing kind of pain?"
"Yeah, that's it. It feels like a truck ran over me."
"Exactly where do you feel it?"
"Well, like here," (chest) "but it sort of shoots out."
"Does it shoot out to your arm?"
"Yeah, this one." (pointing to left arm)

Pain is, among other things, a symptom. In a heart attack, a sudden onslaught of acute chest pain may alert both patient and doctor to the fact that something is distinctly wrong. The kind, location, and extent of that pain becomes a diagnostic aid. Hence the doctor's attempt to pin down the sensation by means of the question and answer technique and by means of adjectives and metaphors.

Not to find the exact nature of the sensation would be bad doctoring, tantamount to overlooking blood spurting from a wound. Not to give accurate answers would be downright foolishness on the patient's part. The fact that the pain involved in a heart attack may initially resemble that of acid indigestion does not mean that we can necessarily afford to rush straight to the medicine cabinet, from the heartburn to the alkalizer, from *situation* to *tactics.* Such a rush for relief, however attractive, might lead straight to the mortuary. Careful attention to descriptive adjectives (assuming the

13

acute pain continues), related to a competent observer, might mean the lesser penalties of a stay in the local cardiac intensive care unit, a reduction in weight, and a ban on cigarettes.

This leads to another observation about pain, one which deserves careful exploration. The linguistic roots of the word are ominous and point to some of the associated emotional undertones that every pain person hears: Latin, *poena*, Greek, *poine*, means "fine" or "penalty." As Job found, to his spiritual dismay, we may have a penalty inflicted on us when we have no idea at all what we did to merit it. In psychogenic pain (that is, pain having no discernible physical cause) we are perhaps engaged in some unexamined, unknown trade within the punishment/penalty area. We are perhaps turning an inner need for punishment into a physical pain. Unlikely as it may sound to non-pain persons, many people relish pain of a physical nature. Physical pain allows them to bury emotional pain.

If the English "pain" and its roots point to punishment, other languages point in similar directions. The French "douleur" and "mal" lead us to "sadness" and "evil"—in sum, affliction. Chinese words are of particular interest, since the written word-forms are themselves descriptive. Chinese writing is ideographic. That is, a symbol is placed on paper as a picture of what is meant. The central symbol for Chinese "pain" words is that of a bed. One is prostrated, laid low, or (again) afflicted and even abnormal. Similar language transactions take place in Hungarian, Russian, and German. The problem of definition and description is not restricted to English-speaking people. Each culture adds to its basic word or symbol the needed qualifying labels. In English we speak of a *head*ache; in French we speak of mal-de-*tete*. Other languages do not define the intruder. They merely confirm what we already know: It is relatively easy to describe pain; it is very difficult to define it, even in medical terms.

Annoying or obnoxious as we may find television commercials, they do help shape our metaphors for everything from cleanliness to godliness, including pain. In the commercials, pain presents itself to us as a *thing,* an entity, belonging roughly to the same league as dirt, bugs, perspiration odor, and tight girdles. If television gives us that message, it also places pain in the general category of things to be done away with, or not to be spoken of in polite society. (Commercials about pain relievers were among the few things that used to amuse me. I viewed them as ridiculous, pompous, and totally inappropriate.) "Pain-as-thing" ranks along with cockroaches, ring-around-the-collar, and other uglinesses, common to everyday human life, but not entirely respectable. Just as no self-respecting housewife (we are told) can put up with stains on the permanent press shirt, so no self-respecting pain person (we are told) ought to put up with pain, whether it is associated with hemorrhoids or headache or constipation.

"Pain-as-thing" does have its attractions. It satisfies many doctors, many sufferers, and many of those who suffer the sufferers, since the concept meets a universal need to put the culprit in its place. "Pain-as-thing" satisfies many in the medical profession, in that pain indicates (sometimes) a physical abnormality, in much the same way that stains on a shirt front may point to sloppy eating habits. Find the cause (sloppy eating habits) and eradicate the thing, hopefully permanently. "Pain-as-thing" also frequently (although sometimes disastrously) satisfies the pain person: Remove the thing and we can go back to work, enjoy sex again, resume life as it was. Furthermore, "pain-as-thing" satisfies many of those who live with the pain person, who, contrary to his or her personal, isolated view, is *not* alone in the world. The people around us also suffer, if only from having to cope with whining, self-pity, irritability, and the other unpleasant, outspread side effects: Grandma has a chronic pain in her neck; as she does so, those in her immediate vicinity may come to regard *her* as a pain in the neck. "Pain-as-thing," then, is an attractive, seductive representation of the intruder. If we can get rid of "it," we can all go about other, more important business. Unfortunately, the idea of "pain-as-thing" is neither accurate in medical terms nor useful in practice. Some pain cannot be removed or eradicated. To look upon such forms of pain as removable, like a piece of trash, or erasable, like a stain, is to delay or deny help to the pain person.

Physiologically, pain is a process, not a thing. Certain nerve fibers transmit, by a combination of electrical and chemical relays, information about a *stimulus* (noxious, if you like). The information goes along to the cerebral cortex of the brain and thence to an ill-defined memory bank in the recesses of the brain itself. As information about the stimulus reaches the cerebral cortex, a sorting-out takes place—*perception.* * (Something's the matter with your hand or your toe or your belly, something that you relate to previous experiences with hands and toes and bellies.) "Pain-as-thing" speaks only to the stimulus. It fails to deal with the procedural problems of perception. But if we are lucky, once we perceive the stimulus, we can take immediate remedial action

---

*I am deliberately oversimplifying here. The neuroanatomy of pain is fascinating, but not everyone is wild about learning new languages. There is still some debate going on in medical journals about the details of the pain process. If any readers wish to enter the jungle of medical jargon to find out about synapses or dorsal roots or the thalamus, I wish them good luck. But it is usually better to let the experts juggle the jargon. Amateur practitioners may lose their footing.

—remove the splinter, buy some corn plasters, or settle in for a case of the twenty-four hour flu.

Whether we are lucky or not, during the pain process something else is going on inside the head. The pain experience, as we perceive it, attaches itself to our past histories of pain. Again, a cruel complication, especially when the causes are blurred or when the pain does not yield to familiar relief measures. Have a headache? Reach for the aspirin. But what if aspirin doesn't work? And what if headaches, in the past, carried other meanings than the one currently being felt?

When we were children, and we all once were, pain associated itself with many other experiences: a spanking or a beating (*Bad* boy! *Bad* girl!); scolding (See? I *told* you not to climb that tree!); being left to the mercies of a strange person in a white uniform sticking needles into us (Now you be *good* while the doctor takes care of you!); and so forth and so on. Perhaps we received a great deal of attention—most of us probably did: "Here, darling, Mommy will kiss it and make it well"

At least part of Grandma's pain in the neck can be traced to the fact that she too was a child once. Her pain gets her a familiar kind of attention, attention she might otherwise not get, and she may well continue to complain, knowing intuitively, if not consciously, that those taking care of her will have to listen. A pattern of *response* to pain gets established early and stays with us. Response to pain is as much a part of the process as the original pain stimulus.

Two personal observations about conscious and unconscious responses to pain. As a child, I discovered how to manufacture very convincing symptoms of a cold and sore throat. So, whenever I had a good book to read and was bored with school, I earned myself a quiet day off, with lots of attention plus lunch in bed. More to the point, however, my earliest memory is that of falling against a chair in the hall and suffering a very painful cut lip. I cannot remember being scolded for bleeding on the rug, but I know now that my parents were away on a trip when it happened. That piece of ancient history, along with some other pieces, helps account for the sense of desolation and abandonment I frequently felt when the pain in my hand flared.

The psychological effects of chronic pain can be devastating, since under certain circumstances the intruder takes complete charge, and pain seems to become a permanent way of life, something like a war without visible end.

Chronic pain is not the only pain with this power—a point that the pain person may wish to reflect upon. Each of us knows something about pain as a way of life. A migraine headache, for example, can usually be described with fair accuracy, but the experience of a migraine remains unshared by those of us on the outside. The migraine sufferer is swallowed up by pain. Although the pain of childbirth is, by its very nature, self-limited and quickly forgotten, the process may absorb a woman's total consciousness. Even a cut finger demands complete attention, if only very briefly.

No one undergoing the intruder's onslaught has much interest, at least for the duration of the attack, in things which normally preoccupy us. To the pain person, nothing could prove less newsworthy than the economic forecast, the campaign for governor, the school budget, or the latest best seller, unless by some happy chance such topics can serve as distractions. Even then, try engaging in light social conversation with a woman in the final stages of labor and see how much attention she has to spare you. For the pain person, whether the assault is acute or chronic, his or her way of life has been altered, be it for a few minutes or for years. Those of us who stand around and wring our hands or try to help frequently cannot even comprehend the language of that way of life, at least not until the pain process subsides or comes to an end or yields to superior forces.

It is important to remember that pain is a way of life, not a "thing"; it is important to remember that all of us (save a very few) have gone through it. So the sense of isolation is, paradoxically, a shared one. And one way in which the outsider can reach the besieged pain person is that of remembrance: What was it like when the dentist hit a nerve? or when the doctor fixed a dislocated joint?

When the invasion is brief in duration (as with the cut finger) the return to more or less normal life is correspondingly rapid, although we usually permit ourselves to bask a little in the loving attention and concern of bystanders. But when the onslaught is prolonged, other and darker effects begin to exhibit themselves. Pain persons, like the dying, live through stages similar to those described by Dr. Elisabeth Kübler-Ross. They deny what they are living in. They get angry and depressed. They grieve. If they are fortunate, they learn what acceptance is. Unfortunately for pain persons, the stages must be lived through repeatedly, because the intruder doesn't die, nor does the pain person, unless the pain is symptomatic of something fatal. The intruder may be repelled successfully on Monday and be back at the gate on Friday, all of which saps energy and will.

The best single definition/description I have found belongs to Dr. T. S. Szasz:

> . . . [A]ll pain is a consequence of the perception of a threat to bodily integrity, where the body is considered to be an object which is separate from and valued by the ego. The determination of the classification of the pain, i.e., whether it is "real" or "neurotic," depends on

the assessment of an observer of the objective reality of
the threat. Pain, whatever its original cause, may come
to take on secondary communicative or symbolic nature, and may persist because of these characteristics.*

Big words. But when slightly revised for the average pain
person and for those around him or her, the definition/de-
scription looks like this:

All pain is the result of what we see to be a threat to
our bodies. We look at our bodies as things belonging
to our inner selves, extensions of *us,* necessary to the
choices and decisions we consciously make. The pain
may be called "physical" (or "organic") or "emotional" (or "psychogenic"). Sorting out the labels is the
job of an outsider, who can tell whether the pain is
fundamentally physical or emotional. Whatever started
the pain—an injury or an emotional crisis—pain itself
may serve as a means of saying something to the outside world: *help!* or pay attention! or here I am! Pain
may even turn into an odd sort of shorthand, into
which we translate all kinds of things that really have
nothing to do with its beginnings. Because we use pain
to say something, and because it works as a shorthand
device, we get accustomed to using it; it becomes a
crutch.

Notice here a spooky correspondence between what I have
termed the "intruder" and what Dr. Szasz calls a "threat,"
and between my "personal territory" and his "bodily integrity."

His description of the after-effects could have been written
about me, as well as about other pain persons I have met and
interviewed. A traveling salesman developed back problems

---

*In *Pain and Pleasure: A Study of Bodily Feelings* (New York: Basic Books, 1957).

because of the amount of time and the number of miles he spent driving. Neurologists found that he had a physical basis for his pain, what is usually referred to as a "slipped disc." A neurosurgeon operated, successfully. But the salesman has recurring problems with his back. He says, "The company has broken my back." Everyone knows the "company" did nothing of the sort. But his perception of pain has reached the shorthand level. He is really saying, "My job and all it entails is back-breaking." And in a real sense, it is. Who is to deny him his metaphor? In a similar sense, a construction worker, disabled by back pain, feels that *his* job "broke his back." After several surgical procedures, he still suffers. He says, "The bones in my back just burn." And who is to deny him his metaphor?

In my case, outside observers (orthopedists, neurologists, and neurosurgeons) also determined that the threat was "real"; but the threat so unnerved me that I needed the help of a psychotherapist. Why did it unhinge me? Because (and I remember saying this to my psychotherapist) my hands were necessary to me, to my mind, to my identity as a teacher and writer. How could I express my ideas or cook or drive to work or do up lecture notes without my hands? The site the intruder attacked was loaded with symbolic possibilities. Much of the work I did in psychotherapy was devoted to getting at the neurotic pain called up by the injured nerve.

I did get a lot of attention and sympathy, which I like just as much as anyone else. I also demanded attention and sympathy. And as time passed, the demand for attention became a part of my way of life. But it had to be the right kind of attention. It had to conform to my personal standards. Mercifully, I cannot see myself as others saw me during the worst of it.

All of which may explain, at least in part, why pain per-

21

sons can be so unattractive, why Grandma has, and is, a pain in the neck. What is most needed is a break in the patterns of feeling and behavior that pain imposes on us, whether they be physical or emotional or a witches' broth of the two.* Surrender to the intruder only prolongs the agony for everyone, including the pain person. Thus it is necessary to know what the intruder really is, how to disarm it, how to live within a besieged fortress.

It might help to take note of the fact that when Irish clans went into battle, the poet-musicians led the way, marching ahead of the soldiers. They were singing; they were labeling, indeed libeling, the enemy with magical musical names and epithets, thereby presumably softening the backbones of the opposition. The poets knew what all of us instinctively know: Identifying and describing the intruder is the way to begin

> By the word "information" we denote all the knowledge which we have of the enemy and his country; therefore, in fact, the foundation of all our ideas and actions. . . . A great part of the information obtained in War is contradictory, a still greater part is false, and by far the greatest part is of a doubtful character. What is required of an officer is a certain power of discrimination, which only knowledge of men and things and good judgment can give.
>
> —*von Clausewitz*

---

*The word "psychosomatic" needs to be brought in here. The word is widely misused, even by physicians. A "psychosomatic" ailment is one with discernible physical damage, but one which is caused by emotional or mental problems. Ulcers, for instance, are commonly classed as psychosomatic, since some life styles and occupations produce ulcer patients. True, there is a diagnosable ulcer; but also true, there are emotional and mental factors that caused the stress that caused the ulcer. "Psychosomatic" should not be confused with "psychogenic." "Psychogenic" means that there is no discernible physical damage; it does *not* mean there is no pain.

2

The Situation, or What's It Like In There?

Each pain person moves inside what he or she perceives to be a highly individualized environment, one bounded by intensely personal limits. To some extent, every human being does the same thing, and pain persons are human beings before, during, and after the intruder's invasion.

Normally, we share with other people many areas of our lives and find common grounds of concern: our sentiments about income taxes, for example, and our worries about the raising of children, "law and order," and the cost of living. With those close to us we share even more intimate concerns, and when all goes well we feel the better for that sharing. But each person's history is unique, since as human beings we come equipped with distinctive characteristics and backgrounds as individual as our fingerprints. At the same time that we like being "together," we jealously cling to "myself." And most of us hang on to our separate identities as if they were money in the bank.

The pain person's human thirst for individuality is greatly enhanced. It's *my* body that hurts, *my* territory that the intruder attacks. It's *me* that suffers, not the doctor or the neighbor, or even the body in the hospital bed next to mine. Nobody else had my childhood. Nobody else has exactly the same genes, the same education, the same hobbies, the same pain experiences, past and present. No X-ray or diagnostic sentence will take these away from me.

The "I'm different" conviction produces unfortunate consequences among pain persons. Primarily, it serves to reinforce the isolating quality of pain. The more we, as pain persons, insist on being unique, different, alone, the more substance we give to that barricade we have to break through if we are to defeat pain. "I'm different" blinds us to the fact that what we, as pain persons, endure is something that is indeed shared by others, if not precisely in the same manner or form or at the same time or to the same degree.

Listen to the kind of conversation that commonly goes on in a physician's waiting room:

> "What time was your appointment?"
> "Two-thirty, and here it is almost three-fifteen."
> "Oh, mine was for two o'clock. . . . Are you here to see Dr. B.?"
> "Yup. I broke my arm about three months ago, and it still isn't right. They sent me here to see if he could do something. What's wrong with you?"
> "Oh, I don't know, exactly. I guess it's arthritis. I have this terrible pain in my hip. . . . I wish they'd hurry up."

And so on. The chatter drifts into comparisons and contrasts of symptoms and doctors, and individual situations emerge and cross-fertilize, so that two individuals unwittingly discover that they move along a common path. It's a pity that they never meet again. The path they briefly move along together is, they will independently find, bewildering, frustrating, and laced with obstacles that they have neither been instructed about nor warned against. But the fact that, out of boredom, restlessness, or irritation, they momentarily share a common concern might alert them to the more important fact that they are not alone, even if their complaints are individual and specialized.

Because such conversations do go on, it is not out of order to construct, from our individual bits and pieces, a hypothetical case history. What happens when the intruder takes charge?

Meet Mr. A.

Mr. A is a pain person. He can be any age we want him to be—let's say he's 45. He hurt his back a few weeks ago (playing tennis, sailing, building a barbecue in the back yard, bowling, changing a tire, or whatever). Apart from the back pain, which has now extended itself to his leg and is beginning to interfere with his daily living habits, he has always been healthy. He played football and basketball in high school, and he never misses the pro games on TV. A bit overweight, of course, but he plans to go on a diet. Cigarettes? Well, yes, he does smoke more than he should. Liquor? Not too much, mind you, but there's nothing like a couple of drinks before dinner to relax a person. His family? Great, just great. No history of heart disease at all.

The doctor's questions and examination may prove a bit embarrassing, when Mr. A limps in to have his back tended to. But Mr. A isn't worried yet. It's just this back pain. He answers the questions to the best of his ability ("It's a stabbing pain") because he honestly wants the pain to be removed. The doctor prescribes some pain medication and advises bed rest. Mr. A goes home. He tries to follow the doctor's orders, but he does have to go to work. The pain pills help, but somehow they don't kill the pain as thoroughly as he assumed they would. The pain is still bothering him. In fact, the more he thinks about his back, the worse it seems to be. So he reappears in the waiting room, a month later, asking that *Something be done.* The doctor, well aware that Mr. A may have a problem in the spinal column, renews the pain pill prescription and refers him to a specialist, usually either an orthopedist or a neurosurgeon.

Another waiting room, after a lapse of perhaps several weeks ("The doctor can see you on May 15th at 4:30 in the afternoon"). The specialist orders some tests (and those too take time to be arranged), asks some more questions, and finally Mr. A gets a definition to pin on his lapel—let's award him a "slipped disc." Another prescription for painkillers. (Note that this process of referral may well have taken quite some time to be completed. Note also that those painkillers may be fairly potent, and that no one has seriously inquired about the "couple of drinks before dinner.") The specialist suggests what is, I think, quaintly called a "conservative" approach: complete bed rest and a heating pad. This is scarcely good news for Mrs. A, who now not only gets to take out the garbage and walk the dog, but also gets to carry trays to the sufferer's bedside, while doing what she normally does around the house or at her job.

Mr. A, fortified not only with the pain pills and his "couple of drinks" but with a label for this back "thing," does exactly as he was told to do. Apart from the pain, he's almost beginning to enjoy lying in bed. The children are more polite than they've ever been, he doesn't have to go to work, and his wife is being very kind to him. Unfortunately, the pain gets no

26

better. Again, the more he thinks about it, the worse it seems. He calls the specialist, and a month later (hospital beds are hard to come by) surgery is performed. The pain rapidly recedes, has stopped, in fact, by the time he is discharged from the hospital, feeling fine, carrying in his pocket a prescription for a *limited* number of painkillers.

When the pain comes back a few months later, Mr. A begins to be anxious. He thinks, "That operation was supposed to cure me, and it didn't." He still enjoys the attention he gets, but somehow there seems to be less of it. His wife shows signs of wear and tear, and the children have stopped being polite. The pain pills have run out. He limps back to the specialist (he cannot walk correctly), who now prescribes physical therapy.

The physical therapist is a delightful and helpful person, but pain limits the treatment. It takes Mr. A several sessions to get his walking gait even somewhere near normal, and his back still hurts. He starts to worry more. What if something went wrong in surgery and they aren't telling him? What if it gets worse? What if it's *cancer?* He notices things he never noticed before: His bad leg looks a little smaller than the other one; he has a twinge in his shoulder; his feet ache. What does it all mean? Another trip to the specialist's office. This time the specialist refers Mr. A to another specialist, probably someone who specializes in neurology or neurosurgery.

Now Mr. A is admitted to a big city hospital, where he is altogether on his own. This time he has a thorough examination, with diagnostic tests he's never been exposed to before. The tests take about a week. His wife only visits him once, because it's the time of the annual PTA fund-raising event. When she visits him, she's nervous and somewhat less than sympathetic. The two of them find little to talk about except the physical examinations, hospital food, and how long it takes the X-ray people to get around to him.

Finally, the test results come in, and the pain specialist tells Mr. A that further surgery is not "indicated." However, some other unrelated problems did show up in the test results. Mr. A's liver has been damaged without his knowing it (those relaxing drinks!); his blood pressure is elevated. And there can be no more painkillers because Mr. A has shown symptoms of withdrawal pangs.

Now Mr. A has been launched into an ocean of unforeseen physical and emotional troubles. All he wanted was help for Lower Back Pain. All he got was more, much, much more, than he bargained for.

How will he respond? If he is like most pain persons, he will feel outraged and helpless. The months of pain have left him in a situation he cannot endure but cannot manage, let alone comprehend. He is angry at the doctors who have failed to help him, at the wife whose attention seems to have drifted away, at his friends who have tactfully deferred to his complaints and no longer ask him to join them for poker, and at fate, or God, or the universe in general. If, by chance, the specialist at the big city hospital had suggested a psychiatric consultation, he's also angry at the psychiatrist: The pain *isn't* in his mind; it's *real.* Doesn't anybody understand?

Although he is probably unaware of what has happened, Mr. A's helpless anger has begun to erode his personality.

Precisely because he is unaware that he has embarked on a way of life allotted to hundreds of thousands of others, he limps around alone in search of a magical cure. He checks out transcendental meditation—no good. He orders a copper bracelet from a mail-order house—no good. He tries faith healing—it doesn't work. He would try acupuncture, save that the idea of needles makes him nervous. As the dreary weeks and months roll on, Mr. A unconsciously slides into the position of a cripple. He has finally started to receive disability benefits (an exhausting victory in itself, but one which officially endorses his self-image). He spends his days in front of the TV. To all intents and purposes, he is no longer Mr. A. The man who loved to play tennis or golf, or to sail, or to fix up the place, or to go bowling, has been replaced by a whining, self-pitying grouch—even, perhaps, what some doctors and laypersons call a "crock." As for his wife, well, their sex life has dwindled away to practically nothing at all (and she may or may not welcome that aspect of pain). She endures his complaints; for her own private reasons, she may even chime in with them. The children go about their own business, as do all his friends. Mr. A is now a member of the society of pain persons, but he doesn't know it.

Not a pretty picture, but a common enough experience.

Many things have conspired to bring about the destruction of Mr. A. Some of them have to do with what I have described as the concept of "pain-as-thing." As long as he cannot—or will not—examine what pain has done to his psyche,* how an intrusive force has driven him into anger and depression, he will continue to park the blame for his condition on any convenient doorstep, the medical profession's, his family's, or his own (his "damned back"). He still thinks of his pain as a "thing," and he cannot see that "it" cannot be excised, like a wart or an ingrown toenail.

But other, less obvious factors have also taken him in hand and led him to his bed. Some of these factors are social and cultural. Like most good American children, he heard over and over again that "As long as you've got your health, you've got everything." It follows naturally that "If you

---

*A nifty catch-all term for "mind," "emotions," "soul," and everything that *isn't* strictly physical. "Psycho-," as a prefix, means emotional or mental. It is not a dirty word, although it frequently is used as one.

don't have your health, you don't have anything." Again, "Good boys don't cry when they fall down and scrape their knees." So? "You mustn't cry, even when you want to scream and beat your head on the floor, assuming you could bend down to do so." That particular bromide, the one about not crying, seems to affect more men than women. As an American rule, women at least are not trained not to yell. They may use up more Kleenex, but they usually don't have to swallow their tears and find the tears turning into corrosive bile.

Mr. A learned other things as he grew up. He broke his leg playing football in high school. He got, as a result, very flattering attention from the cheerleaders, who autographed his cast, and from his family, who waited on him day and night, and even from his teachers, who allowed him to skip homework assignments. He also found out, early on, that his world looks at handicapped people, including those handicapped by pain, as objects of morbid curiosity or distaste. His memory of being an object of attention and flattery, as well as his unconscious assumptions about the way people see him, increases his exquisite perception of pain. He thinks he hates being thought of as an object of anything. He thinks he sees himself as a person. In actuality, he has begun to treat himself as an object. He is going downhill at an ever-increasing rate.

What on earth happened to the ordinary, decent, hardworking individual, proud of himself, enjoying his individuality? He has been transformed. What was once a human being has turned into an ill-tempered snail, all curled up in a very private shell, inaccessible and untouchable.

And, lest we forget, Mr. A could be Mrs. B, young John C, Ms. D, college student E, and the uncounted number of individuals who constitute the alphabetical index of pain.

It is always a grave error to underestimate the social and cultural forces that help to shape our attitudes toward pain. It's bad for the pain person, of course, because he or she badly needs to know what goes into the make-up of individual feelings about the experience. But it's also bad for those on the outside. When they overlook those forces, they fail to comprehend what sorts of pressures are brought to bear on pain persons.

Is another person's pain experience one to be handled as if it were a tragedy? Excessive sympathy and attention are almost as addictive as codeine. People may mean well when they say "Oh, you poor, poor thing!" and "Here, let me do that!" and "Does it feel a little better now, darling?" Yet even the best intentioned sympathy necessarily acts like a magnifying glass when overused. It enlarges pain. It focuses not on the person, but on the intruder.

At the other extreme, excessive dislike or disapproval can work out equally badly; and there are many people who dislike or disapprove of those who express pain. The notion that a stiff upper lip is somehow more attractive or better or more socially acceptable than a quivering one can drive the pain person deeper into isolation. (This particular notion is linked strongly to cultural heritage, incidentally. Some cultures object to screaming a lot more than others.) If sympathy is like a magnifying glass, disapproval is like the wrong end of a telescope. It puts the pain person far, far away, outlawed by social opinions which value fortitude above all. Few outsiders come right out and say that they disapprove of expressions of pain. Instead, they utter ironic platitudes, such as "If you ask me, it's all in her head." An unintentionally accurate observation, even allowing for the fact that nobody asked that it be uttered. As we have already seen, pain *is* in the head, but such oversimplifications are not laughable. The *perception* of pain is just as real to the pain person whose doctors have found no organic cause as it is to the one who has a folder full of X-rays that do show something.

There are other social and cultural attitudes that are fully as unhelpful as excessive sympathy or disapproval. Take the way most people regard that naughty condition called "hypochondria." If all the world loves a lover, all the world shuns the hypochondriac. Yet I am certain that the most stoic personality among us has, at some time or other, suffered attacks of hypochondria. It's all in what we mean by the word. *Stedman's* defines it as "a morbid concern about the health and exaggerated attention to any unusual bodily or mental sensations. . . ." It has also been called "fascinated absorption" with what's going on in the body, with that threat to bodily integrity posed by pain. According to the rule, then, everyone has probably been a hypochondriac, on more than one occasion.

Being "fascinatedly absorbed" with threats to the body is a very common experience. While it is true that professional football players endure a tremendous amount of physical strain, think of a quarterback who has just been rudely pulled down by a 250-pound linebacker: He will be altogether fascinated with his body's condition and with threats of pain and impairment, because his livelihood depends on his throwing arm. For that matter, most of us have been brought up to look upon our bodies exactly as a hypochondriac does. We have been conditioned since infancy to give exaggerated attention to bodily sensations ranging from cuts and bruises to bowel movements. The so-called "hypochondriac" is to a degree exactly like the rest of us, except we'd rather not listen and we'd really rather not be bothered. One expert suggests that we hate in others what we see in ourselves.

Most pain people become, practically speaking, hypnotized by their experiences, whether the pain is organic or psychosomatic or psychogenic. I'll offer my own case as an example. No one could have been more fascinatedly, if not morbidly, absorbed in the experience of pain and threat of impairment than I was, especially in the darker winter of discontent. I was the perfect example of hypochondria. In fact, now that I think of it, "absorbed" seems rather a weak word. I was immersed, coming up for air only when forced to by circumstances. Yet there was clinical evidence of a damaged nerve; the pain was not imaginary.

Perhaps it would be as well if the general public forgot it ever heard of "hypochondria." Doctors can have it as a diagnostic tool, but the rest of us should put it in the same category as ethnic slurs and other obscenities.

One of the single most damaging social and cultural forces that prey on the pain person is the still common public attitude toward psychotherapy and psychiatrists. We show our nervousness about the territory of the mind when we rely on cute terms in talking about it. We refer to "head-shrinking" or the "shrink"; we refer to "crazy doctors" and to "wig-pickers." Although many idealists cherish the belief that psychotherapy now enjoys widespread acceptance by a majority of the population, there are a great many doubting Thomases around, more than we perhaps realize. Furthermore, it's one thing to make smug pronouncements about psychotherapy and its importance. It's quite another thing to find oneself in a hospital as a pain person with a documented physical problem and to hear the specialist suggest a psychiatric consultation. "You mean there's something the matter with my *mind?*" No matter how sophisticated and well-educated the person may be, the suggestion comes as a shock.

Our responses vary widely to the notion that psychiatry can help pain persons, and probably range from outrage through terror to passive obedience. But if we think of psychiatry as something for "crazy" people or people with hangups or delusions, then we have surely allowed ourselves to be brainwashed by the world around us. Whether we are pain persons or not, we need to know why psychotherapy is important in the pain experience. Depression, for instance, cripples just as much as pain does. And long-term pain can cause depression; in fact, it very frequently does. In other words, one needn't be some kind of freak to feel that things are closing in when pain persists. On the contrary, it might even be said that there were something the matter if we weren't depressed. And the person to see for depression is the psychiatrist, or the psychiatric social worker, or at least a doctor who knows something about treating depression.

Look again at Mr. A. He really needn't live in that shell, watching TV all day long. Had he been helped by psychotherapy when he was set adrift on that ocean to sink or swim, he might have been better equipped to manage his anger and depression. He might have found out why he felt as he did and how his emotions helped to shape the shell he now occupies. His picture of himself might be brighter than it is. Whose fault is it that he never got psychiatric help? Some of the fault may lie with the doctors, who perhaps failed to recognize the early warning signals; some of it lies with his own fear of "shrinks"; most of it lies with the world he lives in. The tragedy is that all too often neither he nor his family knows that things might have been otherwise.

And this brings us to a deeper level of social and cultural influences.

We get our messages about pain from all kinds of sources,

from conversations at the dinner table, from the way friends
and families talk about the problem, from memories so well
and thoroughly buried that we don't know they exist. Some
of these messages reflect very, very ancient myths about pain.
(By "myth" I do not mean "fairy tale" or "untruth." A myth
is a way of saying something that cannot find expression in
simple terms.) Volumes have been written about pain myths.
I will point out only three simple myth-equations:

1. Pain =punishment for something we've done
   wrong.
2. Pain =making up for something we've done wrong,
   or for something wrong with the world we
   live in.
3. Pain =something that only grown-ups can handle.

Myths like these are so deep-rooted that we hardly ever think
about them consciously. Nonetheless, they exert a powerful
force on our imaginations. I need scarcely add that imagination is "funny." It takes odd twists and turns, some of which
add curious dimensions to the pain experience.

1983409

Take the pain = punishment one, for a start. We find the
myth quite plainly stated in the biblical story of Adam and
Eve. Because they disobeyed God, they were afflicted: cast
out of the Garden of Eden (a painless state of being), they
must pay a "penalty" for what they did wrong. Adam has
to sweat for a living. Eve must bear her children in "pain"
or "sorrow." God alone knows how many women in childbirth have, over the centuries, had their labor pains inten-
sified by an unexamined, unidentified sense that they are
paying for what was at the time an innocent pleasure. For
Adam's sons, there will always be rocks to break, land to

irrigate, jobs to be won, competition to be endured, pain of a degree as acute as Eve's. (One of my favorites from a fat collection of well-meant but unhappily voiced comments: "I think it's just a sin that you're having so much pain." The connection with Adam and Eve didn't dawn on me for a while, but when it did, I was struck by the enduring power of the pain=punishment myth.)

How does the pain person sense the myth? Well, he or she may in all likelihood feel, or even say aloud, "Why *me?* I haven't done anything to deserve this. I've always tried to be a good person, I've earned my own living, I've paid my taxes, and I've done what I was told to do." The problem here is that nearly everyone is a little uncertain as to his or her own virtue. Hardly a person alive doesn't harbor some guilty secret or other. The sudden onslaught of acute pain may not evoke a sense of guilt; but let the pain continue, and the "What did I do to deserve this?" cry will betray the myth's power. The punishment feeling goes on whether the pain is "organic" or "psychogenic" or "psychosomatic."

The myth having to do with pain as a way of making up for something is a little different from, somewhat more complex than, the pain=punishment one, although the two have certain qualities in common. The term used here is "expiation." We think we, in our liberated twentieth century, have outgrown "expiation." We haven't. It appears and reappears, in all sorts of variations

The oldest variation runs somewhat along these lines: There's a plague, a famine, or a war going on. Obviously, the gods or God are displeased. Something has to be done. We must appease the powers by dumping our social sins onto the head of a victim, or scapegoat, who can usually be identified by a moral, physical, or psychological "abnormality." The scapegoat suffers, perhaps is killed, on behalf of others. In this arrangement, the victim gains a curious peace of mind in being selected for the "job" of suffering. Not only does he or she accept the role, he or she may quite willingly embrace it.

Oedipus was one such victim; his own abnormal pride and vanity had as much to do with his blinding himself as did the fact that he unwittingly killed his father, married his mother, and committed incest. He quite willingly embraced his fate at the end of the play. The Jews in Europe, in the 1930s and 1940s, serve as unforgettable examples of the myth brought up to date. They were made the scapegoats of a sick society, and because they lacked the trademark of "Aryanism" and could therefore be treated as "abnormalities," they were chosen to suffer.

Naturally, no sane contemporary society goes *quite* that far with the expiation routine (perhaps). But the pain person dimly senses that all those healthy people on the outside look askance at his or her experience, as if to say, "There, but for the grace of God, go I." Pain singles out individuals, cuts them out of the herd, brands them. Sometimes pain persons do embrace the idea that they are "suffering" for some cosmic purpose; sometimes they gain satisfaction and comfort from that idea. More frequently, however, their pain makes them "abnormal," and the outsiders who deal with them use them as scapegoats.

As we have already observed, Mr. A does not live alone, even though he has curled up in his shell. It is safe to assume that Mrs. A has some problems of her own. So do his friends. So do his doctors.

Mrs. A, for instance, has some guilt feelings that may have nothing whatsoever to do with her husband's back problem. Here she is, stuck with an invalid but still not ready to resign from the human race, as he is attempting to do. When her husband's pain did not yield to medical treatment, the odds are that she was fully as angry and depressed as he. But she has more freedom than he does. Depending on what their life together has been, a good many different options present themselves to her. One of them, of course, is to make him the scapegoat for the kind of life they now must live, a kind of life full of difficult problems and choices.

"If it weren't for him and his back, I could. . . ." Any number of concluding phrases come to mind.

"I could" repaper the dining room. We must not forget that pain costs money, that health insurance and Social Security benefits do not quite add up to enough money to live according to the old ways.

"I could" have a little attention and sympathy for myself. When pain persons get all the attention being handed out, those around them feel angry and resentful, then guilty about feeling that way. Should a pain person enjoy the attention, the situation grows very sticky.

"I could" have a little fun. And fun includes sex. Perhaps Mr. A doesn't care about sex anymore. Mrs. A may not necessarily think of herself as ready for the trash heap at the age of forty-two. It needn't be assumed that she will go out in search of extracurricular sexual adventure, but such things have happened. And guilt probably follows.

What goes on in that household merely brings the old myth up to date. Mrs. A, knowing unconsciously that the situation is not of her husband's making, but resenting it and harboring guilt feelings, transfers the resentment and guilt to him. She displaces her own burden by placing it on his back. One of two consequences usually ensues. Mr. A, neither strong enough nor feisty enough to tell her to get off his back, endures his role of victim with bewilderment and enhanced pain; or he secretly relishes the scapegoat role, thereby intensifying the hold that pain already has on him. As for friends and doctors, they too participate in the ritual. The friends are guiltily glad that it was A, not they, who was singled out for the intruder's attentions.

As for doctors, it really does bother them that they cannot help him. A few may even unconsciously blame him for not getting well: Haven't they done everything modern medicine can do? One psychiatrist refers to pain persons like Mr. A as examples of "referred" pain—that is, specialists in one field cannot cure the pain, so they "refer" A and his pain along to someone else. What they are really "referring" is their own frustration. Mr A carries that burden for them.

The third myth equation, whose origins are also buried from sight, has to do with pain as part of growing up, and the best indication that the myth is alive and flourishing is the common epithet "cry baby!" In Western nations, we are likely to read about primitive tribes and their "initiation" rites as if we, as highly civilized people, had grown beyond that sort of barbaric nonsense. We don't circumcise twelve-year-old boys, at least, not as a rule. We don't isolate a twelve-year-old girl in the jungle when she first begins to menstruate. We don't subject youngsters to physical pain (to be endured without flinching) before we allow them to vote. We are "beyond" that.

But look at "cry baby!" Its implications are obvious. When we respond to the perception of pain by crying, it means we haven't yet reached an age at which pain responses can be suppressed. Adults ought to manage pain better than children do. Take what happens in the local hospital's Emergency Room. The grown-up who suffers a cut severe enough to warrant treatment tries very hard not to cry. (Wincing is,

I think, permissable, so long as it doesn't interfere with the doctor's stitch-making.) A sobbing adult, whether male or female, is not looked kindly upon by anyone, doctors, nurses, or fellow-inmates. On the other hand, a child who sobs or screams is usually given all sorts of tender, loving care. It's all right for babies to be "cry babies," but not for grown-ups.

This myth affects the pain person in ways the outsider may never perceive at all; it also affects the pain person in ways he or she does not always recognize. The experience of pain, of whatever variety, brings with it a sense of either violent or gradual transition from one level of living to another, from health to non-health, from "okay" to "terrible." The pain person, all alone, like a freshman on the first day at high school, is forced into a brand-new, mysterious country, with all sorts of bewildering rules and regulations. The world of hospitals, for instance, does not belong to the pain person; it belongs to the intruder. Hospital tests can be humiliating and the personnel administering them as callously indifferent as a drill sergeant initiating recruits into the army. The doctors may look like gods or seniors.

By the time a pain person is discharged from the hospital, he will have either passed or flunked the initiation into the pain world. He may have adapted himself to the hospital regime very well, no complaints or questions at all. Or he may have been a "bad" boy. A psychiatrist comments: "Most hospital personnel really appreciate the chronic depressed patient. Those are the people who don't make waves. They just sit quietly. It's difficult to get doctors and nurses to recognize that all that withdrawal and willingness to be cooperative can be a signal that something is wrong."

So much for the "good" pain person. What about the "bad" one, the one who does moan and groan and yell? A surgeon comments: "The personnel don't like the pain patients who complain. They can get very puritanical about giving drugs, for instance." Whichever way it goes, the initiation is in itself painful. But supposing Mr. A accepts the rites of medical procedures without complaint. What happens? Has he reached a new level? No. He gets sent home, sent back, as it were, to the old level. He no longer really belongs there, but he can't stay in the medical world. On the other hand, he's been initiated. The myth within which he grew up turns out to be a "Catch 22."

Apart from the myths, there are people with whom the pain person must deal. They can help and they can hinder, without necessarily knowing what they are doing. We have already noted the damage that excess sympathy can do. Families and friends, trying to be helpful, can, in actual practice, hinder.

Then there are doctors. Discussions about how to tell a good doctor from a bad one take us nowhere in particular, because the doctor-patient relationship is a very complex one, depending as much on the patient as on the doctor's training and skill. (I know a woman who has complete confidence in a gynecologist who refers to all his patients as "girls"; the woman is an intelligent, fully qualified professional, and she is forty years old. I would have walked out of his office in disgust.)

Doctors, like families and friends, can help and they can hinder. Their own attitudes and concepts of pain have much to do with their ability to treat pain persons. If they hold rigidly to the "pain-as-thing" concept, they may be as baffled in trying to treat the "thing" as is the patient. I am told on good authority that fewer and fewer doctors now cling to that conceptual relic of the past. Yet some doctors, for whatever private reasons, seem to want to stay as far away from

41

pain as possible. They keep themselves as free as they can from the pain way of life, armed with the unchallengeable assertion that they should not be involved emotionally, because to become so would damage their clinical objectivity. In the presence of doctors like these, the pain person feels bewildered and rejected. He or she does not know that doctors, like pain persons, have their hang-ups. "The doc didn't seem to care at all. Maybe I didn't explain it right."

Not enough has been written about the pain person's state of mind, and consequently many doctors fail to spot the potentially lethal factors of pain, that is, fear, anger, and depression. The process of pain and the pain person cannot be disentangled, a fact not always apparent to the medical profession or to the public at large. The best doctors for pain persons are those who make an effort to get help to the total hurt—physical and emotional—not just to the back or the shoulder or the hip. Where all the best doctors live and practise, I don't know. I know a few of them, but I also know some who were less than the best. I even encountered a few who truly scared me. For instance, one doctor carefully explained to me that there was no hope at all for my right hand. By the time he had finished his explanation, I felt that I had no hope for life.

Doctors, whether they like it or not, are part of the situation within which pain persons must live. The more they understand that they cannot place themselves above and beyond the pain process, the better off we shall all be. The pain person needs all the help available. It's up to the pain person to take the help offered. It's up to the doctor to keep his own attitude toward pain in order and to offer appropriate help.

At this point it might be well to look at the subject of what is called the "pain threshold." A lot of loose talk about the subject goes on, even in medical journals. Researchers make pontifical statements about "high" and "low" thresholds, as if pain could be measured on a thermometer. It is, in the market place, commonly assumed that women have a higher pain "threshold" than men, because of their biological experience of menstrual cramps and childbirth, although how these things can be measured, except by subjective remarks made by women, I cannot imagine. On the other hand, and almost at the same time, it is asserted that women have a lower "threshold," because they cry more than men. Women say that men don't know what pain *is;* men say that women can't take *real* pain. A stand-off.

When it comes to facts and figures, "pain threshold" is nothing more dramatic than the point at which a "noxious" stimulus is perceived as being "painful." Social and cultural influences have a lot to do with such levels of perception. But some studies show that both men and women perceive a pin prick as painful at about the same time—that is, under laboratory conditions, using willing volunteers.

In ordinary life, the situation is quite different; the specimens have been contaminated by their own histories. Each individual, male or female, brings into the pain experience a lot of personal prejudices, and only rarely is the *non*-volunteer experience willingly undergone. Grown men have cried at the sight of a needle; grown women have paid no attention at all to the same needle. Then again, in real life, some nurses and doctors are ham-handed when it comes to administering needles. Fear has a lot to do with the pain "threshold." If you're sure, on the basis of past experience, that something is going to hurt, it certainly will.

What we, as lay persons, usually mean when we speak from a safe distance about the pain "threshold" is something called pain "tolerance," and here there are gaps created by differences in age, sex, and social and ethnic backgrounds. Infants tolerate much more pain than we think they can, or ought to. (So much for "cry baby!") Men, especially clean-cut, brave Western types, can usually tolerate more pain than women, although I wonder about the clinical findings, since they all seem to be based on experiments involving 28 healthy American college students, all of whom volunteered for the test. (Where are the 28 non-healthy, non-volunteer, non-college students?)

American Indians who have been brought up to believe that Indians can stand more pain than non-Indians show a higher level of pain "tolerance" than do control groups of assorted backgrounds. Since, in many Far Eastern cultures, to react to pain aloud is to disturb other people, it may be assumed that a scream of "I can't take it any more!" is bad form; it may therefore be assumed that, among Far Eastern peoples, the pain "tolerance" level is higher than it is among Americans. In any event, when we talk about pain "thresholds" it is well to be sure what we are talking about.

The pain person lives in a world he or she did not create, a world that intrudes much as does the intruder. That world consists of, in no particular order of importance, such influential factors as: transportation, buildings, jobs, parties, leisure activities, newspapers and TV, restaurants, politics, bureaucracies, and anything else anyone wishes to think of. We might learn, from the pain person's perspective, how these elements of daily life affect the special experience he or she is moving through.

Transportation. How does a man or woman with a bad back drive a car? Few automobiles are constructed with driver's seats that are not bad for someone with lower back pain. In fact, only the deluxe, expensive cars provide someone like Mr. A with the kind of support his back requires. In this regard, as in others to follow, it might be noted that pain as a way of life is expensive. And not only in medical bills. So, driving a car is out. Mr. A and his fellow-sufferers are better off sitting at home.

Buildings. Architects seem to wish to make trouble for pain persons, as well as for all other handicapped people. To the normal, healthy individual, nothing could be more attractive to the eye than one of those gleaming plate glass doors at the new Post Office, the bank, or the high-rise office building. The pain person knows what those doors can mean to the handicapped. What does Mr. A do? He asks his wife to do the errands. It hurts his back when he tries to wrestle with a heavy door.

Jobs. Naturally, if one is applying for a job, an application form must be filled out, and on that form are certain questions. Any physical limitations? Suppose that the pain person answers honestly and says "no lifting of heavy weights," "no sitting in the same chair all day," "no drill press operation," "no typing." Who will hire that pain person? Some companies might, but a lot of others might not.

Parties. These are a bit difficult to take, not only because the pain person remembers well how parties used to be, but because a pain person is a social liability. Pain persons either talk about their pain, in which case they throw the party into depression, or they suffer in conspicuous silence, in which case, too, they throw the party into depression. How does one manage at a party, when the chair one is sitting in is: a) so overstuffed that a Mr. A thinks he'll never get out of it without a derrick; b) so near the floor that only a derrick will move the body; or c) so far from the center of interesting conversation that all conversation, which might prove distracting and therefore allay pain, is out of earshot? The next party invitation may well be sulkily declined. The wife or husband or friend may not like it, but that's how the party way goes.

Leisure activities. Almost all of the traditional ones are beyond reach. Hunting and fishing? Tennis and golf? Touch football and sandlot baseball? Bridge and poker? Tiddlywinks? Anything that requires use of the pain person's personal pain muscles is out, so that many ordinary leisure activities are impossible dreams. Increasing popular emphasis on the "creative" use of leisure time does not help at all. The pain person has more leisure time than do most people. That's one of his or her problems.

Newspapers and TV—or, as we say nowadays, the "media." These are, like narcotics, addictive, but they do give limited access to the world outside. They are channels through which the pain person learns what goes on. People out there are doing great things, winning medals, defeating evil, making a "significant" contribution to humanity, discovering a vaccine, uncovering a scandal, or solving the energy crisis. To a person in a snail shell, most of the word received from the outside says, "You are a non-achiever." Hard news, for an ex-achiever. Soap operas don't hurt quite so much.

Restaurants. I have eaten in quite a few, in recent years, and almost none of them are geared to help the pain person. The chairs are poorly designed. The service is slow (and when something hurts, speedy attention is welcome). If food can take the mind off pain, it should be forthcoming. People at adjacent tables are laughing and drinking and enjoying themselves. The pain person has little to laugh about, less to drink, and nothing to celebrate.

Politics. Pain persons might get excited about politics if

46

politicians had anything to do with where they are. In politics, every candidate has something to say about health insurance, welfare, and senior citizens, the aged, and the poverty-stricken. Somehow all the disadvantaged categories get lumped together, with pain persons tossed in, willy-nilly. The lumping process, like the design of automobile seats, seems almost to have been manufactured to put pain persons into limbo. Being categorized as part of a lump can be remarkably effective in shoving a person back into a shell.

As for bureaucracy, probably nothing more needs saying, as all of us, pain persons and outsiders, have taken our knocks. Everyone can join Mr. A and his fellow-sufferers. But bureaucratic idiocies reinforce the pain shell. They turn the person into a thing and enhance the fallacy of "pain-as-thing." If the IRS conducts an audit on a normal person's tax return, that particular "noxious" stimulus is painless compared to what the pain person undergoes when the bureaucrats sharpen their pencils over a disability claim. As the financial burden of pain grows heavier and heavier, the ugly word "welfare" looms on the horizon. Being relegated to "welfare" destroys anyone's self-image. But these things happen, even in the greatest country on earth. (While I was waiting, for something like twelve months, for the Social Security Administration to grease its creaking wheels, so that my disability claim could be processed, I computed that, had I been without husband or family, I would indeed have been on "welfare.")

In sum, the world the pain person lives in is not constructed to help those who must experience pain as a way of life. Neither, except under special circumstances, is the pain person. Our world, and our self-images, were designed to reflect the needs and wishes of bright, healthy types. If we find ourselves living under the constant assault of pain, we cannot expect much in the way of help from our environment.

But:

> It is, at all times, only conjecture or guesses at truth which we have to act upon. This is why differences of opinion are nowhere so great as in War, and the stream of impressions acting counter to one's own convictions never ceases to flow. Even the greatest impassibility of mind is hardly proof against them, because the impressions are powerful in their nature, and always act at the same time upon the feelings.
>
> —*von Clausewitz*

3

The Problem,
or What's Really Going On?

U ncovering the identity or the name of the intruder is
    one thing. Outlining the problem created by it is
another. Random poking around in the situation of a pain
person generates a good deal of heat but not necessarily
much light. For instance, to every statement made about the
elements that go to make up the situation must be added
qualifiers and disclaimers and exceptions: "sometimes,"
"perhaps," or "usually." Because each pain person is an
individual, not a volunteer for a clinical experiment, each
pain experience differs either a little or a lot from every other
one. Pain persons, their doctors, and their families and
friends do not always notice or understand the variations.
Everyone assumes that all migraines, like all ingrown toe-
nails, produce predictable effects. But headaches and toe-
nails belong to people.

Lower Back Pain, commonly abbreviated in medical literature as LBP, is probably the single most common form of
persistent pain, along with headache and, for women, what

is genteelly referred to as Pelvic Pain. Yet LBP looks very different to different people. It looks like one thing to a potato farmer, who originally got damaged by a back-hoe, who is self-employed, whose wife holds down a full-time job at a shirt factory. It looks like something else to a filing clerk, who originally got damaged in an automobile accident, whose husband is holding down a job and going to night school, who has Blue Cross and two small children. Again, LBP looks like something else to a well-to-do executive, who originally got damaged in a boating mishap, whose wife plays golf at the country club, whose company has excellent medical coverage for him.

These three LBPs belong to people who move in distinctly separate circles. Their worlds revolve in orbits that do not touch each other. The farmer, the clerk, and the executive have perhaps only one thing in common—their pain. They could talk about the way of life they're now engaged in; they could share their experiences and their symptoms. But if they chanced to meet in a hospital day room, they wouldn't want to watch the same TV programs.

Identification of the problem, then, must begin with the assumption that there is a seemingly infinite number of variables to be accounted for.

To put it mildly indeed, the pain person finds it extremely difficult to identify his or her problem in isolation; again, a cruel irony, since isolation goes hand in hand with pain. Fundamentally all that most (but not all) pain people want out of life is for the pain to go away. (One pain person said, "I remember wishing I had cancer. You know why? There's an end to cancer.") The urgently felt need to get rid of pain quite literally blurs the vision, since the intruder looks much larger to the pain person than it does to those on the outside. When the pain keeps right on going, the besieged person cares less and less about its original causes, while the doctors continue to concentrate on trying to find and eliminate the causes. Pain persons might diagram "pain-as-thing" one way, while doctors might diagram "it" otherwise:

Doctor's view: Patient's view:
D-L stands for disease or lesion, lesion being a
medical catch-all word for wound or injury. PA
stands for pain.

The gap between these two pictures of pain's place in an individual scheme of things makes for some awkwardness in communication. In the first place, doctors, just like everyone else, get very frustrated when they can't do what they know they're expected to do. Assume, for instance, that the pain is psychogenic, keeping always in mind that psychogenic pain is as "real" as is the organic or psychosomatic kind. The doctors cannot find a disease or lesion. Hence they may conclude that there is *no* small circle PA. How can there be, if there's no discernible large circle D-L? The patient sees an entirely different image. He or she perceives the large circle PA; he or she wants it taken care of, and the hell with the small circle D-L, whether it exists or not. Some friction will surely result.

Or assume that there is a disease or lesion, but that it cannot be treated medically or surgically. Much as everyone hates to admit the fact, some forms of the intruder are, at least for the time being, beyond the technical reach of the medical profession. ("They said they could operate on one vertebra, but not on all five. So they gave me a body brace and sent me home.") Under these circumstances, doctors may become just as unhappy as their patients.

If doctors and patients look at the pain experience through differing lenses, a similar visual discrepancy affects the pain person's family and friends. It takes a long time for those on the outside to understand that pain can *in itself* constitute a disease or lesion; the intruder can in fact be a plague, can set in motion habits that in turn create lesions. A pain person with LBP may develop some odd posture and a defensive walking gait, thus developing lop-sided shoulder muscles and corns on the toes. Persistent pain spells out the need for a different kind of physical life. It is not, to the individual, an appendage to something else. It can become everything.

So the *image* of the pain experience provides one dimension of the problem. One should never underestimate the power of an image. Movie audiences vomited during "Rosemary's Baby"; students of literature find themselves unable to cope with the poetic image, in Dante's *Inferno,* of Count Ugolino, doomed eternally to gnaw his son's head. The image of persistent, unending pain is, to a pain person, far more frightening than non-pain persons, except for a gifted few, understand.

Another dimension is so self-evident that we frequently overlook its importance. Pain comes in two sizes. It is either a short-term assault (acute) or a long-term one (persistent or chronic). Doctors—and their patients—have little difficulty in dealing with short-term pain, even when it is severe. Surgical and medical measures can tide the short-term pain person over, until such time as the disease or lesion has been healed, or until death puts a stop to everything. The causes of acute pain are almost always obvious.

But every outsider has difficulty in dealing with long-term pain. Perhaps we have all been so brainwashed by the "pain-as-thing" fallacy that our frustrations come to a boil when we confront the grotesqueness of persistent pain. As for pain persons, they often do not know how to pin the proper label on long-term pain. For one thing, they too have been brainwashed by the same fallacy. They have also been conditioned to believe that all pain is, *or ought to be,* short-term. From the inside, persistent or chronic pain usually feels just like acute pain. Furthermore, everyone's vocabulary is unhappily hooked to the terminology properly belonging to short-term, acute pain.

An example: the word "burning." As I said in the Prologue, it seemed to me that my hand was on fire. A useful diagnostic metaphor, since "burning" locates the problem for the doctor; different lesions produce different sensations, as do different kinds of nerves. But the metaphor "burning" is actually far more closely related to acute pain experiences than it is to persistent pain. Had I in fact accidentally touched the palm of my hand with an object hot enough to burn, I would have experienced acute, short-term pain, which would in turn have yielded to treatment (ice-cold water and some pain medication to deaden the sensation while the burn healed). There was no object, no barbecue grill at all. However, "burning" was the only word I knew that in any way described the sensation. My vocabulary was severely limited by my own past history, and all who suffer from persistent pain are similarly limited.

The catch here—that is, the limitations that govern our vocabulary of pain—has to do with something more complex than an ordinary, everyday communication gap. The pain person wistfully clings to an inadequate, but heartfelt, conviction that all pain should be short term. Our word choices, then, betray the terrible truth that we simply do not know what to do about persistent pain. As the lady said, cancer would, on the whole, seem preferable. The prospect of there being no end to the experience is so devastating that all but the most determined personality can easily be reduced to a whine and a whimper. And if such a statement seems extravagant, I can only assert that it is not. Yes, some pain persons *do* kill themselves, either in a single act or by degrees, with an overdose or with alcohol.

A second dimension of the problem, then, is one of language, of words and descriptions having to do with the duration of the pain assault. Insiders and outsiders need to be freed from false and misleading expectations revealed in what we say. (I must add that I have no idea how to get around the language barrier.)

A third dimension is connected to the second. Somehow, both pain persons and those around them need to find some way of measuring the quality and quantity of the pain experience. True, thermometers don't help; nor do many of our subjective observations ("Ooh! It hurts a lot!"). Doctors need measurements for obvious reasons, like the ones sketched in the dialogue in Part I. But pain persons and their families also need measurements, if only because the pain person must learn to distinguish between the bearable and the unbearable. A surprising amount of pain is bearable, despite what some pain persons think and say. A modest effort at honesty can effectively cut the intruder down to size. Besides, doctors have their own techniques for measurement. When pain persons use inaccurate yardsticks, no one is necessarily deceived except themselves, and treatment becomes the more difficult.

Measuring pain levels does pose some dangers, since the act of measurement invites us to get out the magnifying glass, to concentrate on the "thing" instead of the problem. In our hypochondriac moments, we love to measure in exquisite detail and we develop great skill in making fine distinctions. The whole effort may easily deteriorate into "show and tell time." Here the pain person needs a certain degree of detachment, a means of stepping outside the situation. Providing that means may prove difficult, however; and when the pain person is absorbed by the experience, detachment may not seem possible. Outsiders' observations can help. For instance, it might have helped Mr. A to measure his pain had his wife said, when the time was right, "You managed the stairs a lot better today than you did yesterday." Had she said this, and had he heard and digested the observation, he might have found a yardstick.

How much pain can we really tolerate, without screaming? For how long? Under what circumstances?

Back to my "burning." The sensation took different forms. Once I became consciously aware of the differences, I made up a personal numerical scale by which to make measurements. I didn't do so in order to impress or even help my doctors. I did so as an act of self-protection. My scale started at what I called Level 1 (faint "burning," hardly qualifying as pain at all, except that it was annoying and unceasing). Levels 4–6 (a "jabbing" kind of "burning," and if the two adjectives seem oddly paired, so be it) amounted to flares of pain, superimposed on Level 1's constant. Level 9 (the barbecue already mentioned) was so severe that the slightest breath of air passing over my skin was virtually unendurable.

Quite deliberately, I reserved Level 10 for future reference. The general idea seems to have been that "It might be worse, but it isn't yet." The hypothetical Level 10 made Level 9 occurrences easier. On reflection, I think the hidden benefits of my personal scale made it possible for me to keep going. Had I ever been faced with a real, live Level 10 pain, I probably would have killed myself. Fooling myself? Clearly so. But in pain as in war, some forms of deception prove useful.

We still have not examined a loosely affiliated, yet troublesome, aspect of the problem. There are some *non*-pain persons who are not part of the fighting forces, but who for various reasons make life difficult for those who are. Then there are pain persons who, for other reasons and in other ways, make the dimensions of the problem fuzzy and indistinct.

The first group is composed of those who have noticed that pain pays. It pays psychologically, as we have seen: When under assault, the pain person gets sympathy, tender loving care, and a seductive opportunity for self-indulgence. But pain also pays in the coin of the realm—in dollars and cents. Ask any insurance claims adjuster.

"Whiplash" qualifies as the handiest and most notorious specimen for analysis. It's in the nature of the the intruder that initial reports of damage usually get taken at face value. "Whiplash," since it can produce persistent pain, has a lot of face value, if incurred under the correct circumstances. I do not mean to imply that there is no such thing as a bona fide whiplash injury. However, there are a good many nonwhiplash non-injuries. In any event, whether consciously or unconsciously, the whiplash pain person knows good and well that he or she stands to benefit from pain. And there are such people as hangers-on or camp followers in the great wide world of pain. Consider the following:

> "This pain is really killing me." Rubbing the neck vigorously. "It's a stabbing pain, like right here." Pointing. "It never lets up." Moving the head around, looking at the office decor. "This is a really nice place you've got here, doctor. I like the way it's laid out." Dropping a cigarette lighter, bending over to pick it up. "Oh, by the way, did they tell you I've filed a suit against the driver of the car? Well, let me tell you. . . . " Turning the head to light a cigarette.

The non-pain, non-whiplash person betrays himself as a role-player. How severe is his pain? Not very.

There are people who manufacture major pain out of minor twinges. Insurance companies settle claims or pay benefits, and miraculously the "pain" evaporates. The truth is that quite a lot of pain evaporates when money is applied to the afflicted place. For my part, I wish non-pain persons would find another line of work. They interfere with me and others like me. They not only use up too much of my doctors' time, they present a fraudulent portrait of the authentic pain person.

The second group of interferers—these are genuine pain persons—are equally unhelpful. These are the passive prisoners of the intruder. They are the pathetic people who have given up, utterly succumbed, who don't give a damn about themselves or anyone else. They use up others' time, energy, and money. Passive prisoners find it safer, on the whole, to stay where they are, to let other people wait on them, to watch TV all day every day. They fear the risks involved in fighting back, even while they suffer. Passive prisoners closely resemble the prisoners of war who dutifully obey their captors' orders. By staying out of trouble, they think they can outwait the war. They can't. Persistent pain, as an intruder, does not get defeated by a liberating army. There is no liberating army.

These two groups—the camp followers and the well-behaved prisoners—do not really understand what their activities (or non-activities) do, not only to the front-line troops, but to the general public's understanding of the battle. Mr. A, for instance, has the right to remain silent in his snail shell. But as long as he stays silent and refuses to fight the intruder, he drags the rest of the pain population back. When outsiders look at him, feel sorry for him, think of him as bearing up bravely (while he is in reality doing nothing of the sort), they get the idea that passivity is the ideal response to chronic pain. It isn't ideal at all.

So it is not the pathetic soul, sweetly grimacing from the bed of pain, who represents pain as a way of life. Rather, it's the soul who decides to move, to test alternatives, to fight back, who best represents the way. (I am, of course, not talking here about terminal cancer patients. They make up a special group of pain persons, and their pain, while it too is a way of life, is better treated as acute pain.) One mid-western lady had arthritis of a pain level never seriously tested. She spent most of her days on a hospital bed in her living room. From there she exercised a tyranny over her family that reduced them to slavery, all the while smiling sadly. Her friends thought her terribly gallant. Her "sweetness" deceived them. If the camp follower is not a saint, neither does the passive prisoner deserve a halo.

Given the jumble of material that must be accounted for in any delineation of the pain problem, the old-fashioned concept of the pain process has decided limitations. Diagrammatically, that concept looks like:

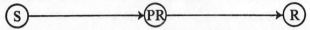

S = Stimulus: the blade of a sharp knife cuts into the skin of the thumb; some nerve fibers send a signal to the brain, thus evoking

PR = Perception; the sensation sent by the nerve fibers is sorted out from other sensations and identified as to location and type; the sensation links up with other, previous sensations of the same sort, gathering up the past into the present, and thus determining

R = Response; the complexities of perception complicate the response; there need be no obvious connection between the stimulus and the response; response includes not only action (running cold water on the cut thumb) but emotions, ranging from mild annoyance to other, deeper feelings, sometimes largely unrecognized.

This, like all other diagrams, including those in medical publications, fails to deal with the individuality of the pain experience, although in the perception and response areas even a diagram allows for differences of opinion.

Reflect again on the potato farmer, the file clerk, and the executive. These are three different human beings, with little in common. To some degree, they live in the same way of life (LBP); but to a far greater degree, they live far apart. The diagram needs adjustment:

Farmer: Clerk: Executive:

Redrawing the diagram frees us to add some much needed extras. Once we enclose the stimulus-perception-response inside the skins of three human beings, we are able to enclose other pertinent information about the pain process.

The pain person's *personality:* given to extended bouts of hypochondria? highly dependent on other people? the eternal pessimist? dull, unresponsive? having, or lacking, a sense of humor? The pain person's *job:* demanding and rewarding? dreary and underpaid? appealing to a "workaholic"? part of the pain person's self-image? The pain person's *family and friends:* their attitude towards pain? the family's history of pain? love pain or loathe it? coddle it or curse it? The pain person's *sex life:* pain is a way out? an extension of the "Not now, darling, I have a headache" motif? pain affects whose sex life? and why? The pain person's own *history of pain:* pain in childhood? an abused child? rewards and punishments for pain in the past? secondary gains from being ill or being hurt? The pain person's *physical and financial condition:* physical factors needing to be accounted for? levels of physical stress that can be endured? financial security or insecurity? gains or losses?

And, of course, we have to add other factors properly belonging to the outside; these are things the pain person has digested without ever having tasted them. What does the *world* he or she lives in think about him or her and about pain? What do his or her *doctors'* attitudes say? What are the *myths* carried around his or her neck? These bits of information make up the pain person's individuality as much as do the other things comprising a case history.

Now the diagram of the pain experience looks like:

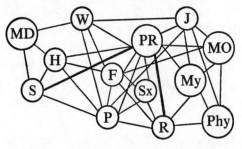

This more complicated diagram (the lines go in all directions as various factors affect each other) allows us to admit into the pain process the many influences that do not at first glance seem to have anything to do with, say, the initial stimulus. The more that is left out, the more distorted the picture of the problem. We can't leave out the doctors; we can't leave out money or sex or personal history. We can't even leave out a husband's or wife's or parent's history of pain, since such histories shape the attitudes toward persistent pain that the pain person must live with.

Each pain person fits into the larger circle, but each individual must draw and color in his or her own smaller ones. A pain person remarks, "I had the good fortune to have had a father who wrote his mother every week, telling her the family news. My grandmother kept those letters, which, after her death and my father's, went to my mother. Those letters contain a running history of my childhood. They gave me a chance to see what my experiences of pain really were. I got to find out what kind of pain I had as a child."

But now that we have a nice, neat diagram of the problem to play with, we still aren't free from pain. Those small circles—especially the one labeled "history"—are not engraved in marble. Our histories of pain keep right on going, as do clocks and calendars. Human beings are not diagrams. Even occurrences like perception and response, which experts think they can measure, cannot be considered as unchanging, in part because each skirmish with the intruder adds something to perception, as well as to response. A second sprain of the same ankle, for example, begets an experience of pain that includes memory of the first sprain.

Since pain is a *way,* not a thing, we can expect to find some mileage markers along the route. Some of the markers are easy enough to spot: doctors' appointments, tests, operations, treatments, and so on. Others may not be so obvious. These are inner, personal markers. How do we feel as we move along?

Emotional mileage markers more closely resemble pages in a diary than they do something put up by the highway department. One day the pain person may feel relatively cheerful (an article in the newspaper announces a "breakthrough" in the treatment of something or other); the next day may bring on a fit of depression; the next, unexpected rage and despair. States of mind swing back and forth, according to levels of pain and other factors. If a pain person were to draw up a personal diagram like the one above, he or she would have every day to add more small circles or to change their color and size. And each new insight about pain —its impact, its severity, or its threat—would need to be drawn in.

Although the stages cannot be staked out in a nice, clear-cut linear progression, they can be subjects for discussion. Anger is one mileage marker. So is denial. (Unlikely as it seems, denial of pain does exist.) Depression, as we already know, is an integral part of the persistent pain way. Then there's something called "acceptance," a state of the psyche that comes in more than one variation and must be examined with great taste and discretion. These stages sometimes mix and mingle, one good reason the "mileage marker" label has its flaws. But they may be disentangled and looked at, just so long as we remember that in actual experience they are woven together.

Denial

What comes to mind immediately, when we talk about denial of pain, is an extinct society, the Spartans of ancient Greece. Spartans were brought up to deny pain, because they were brought up to be the world's greatest warriors. The Spartan mother told her sons, as they went off to battle, to come back either carrying their shields or lying on them. No walking wounded at all. (Well, perhaps technically *some* walking wounded, but definitely no walking *defeated* wounded.) The ancient Spartans may be gone, but they have quite a few spiritual cousins still around. Native Americans traditionally showed, still show, Spartan qualities. Politely bred Far Eastern peoples in some societies probably also qualify as Spartans. So do all those who maintain the proverbial stiff upper lip.

Pain specialists don't see much of contemporary Spartans; since Spartans deny pain, they rarely consult doctors. But we can learn something from them. What they seem able to do is to control their *responses* and thereby perhaps even their perception of pain. How can they possibly control perception? As the diagram shows, perception is in part influenced by myths and by the world in which we live. The same thing goes for response. The myths of the ancient Spartans, like those of their latter-day counterparts, placed great value on non-response, and non-response in turn alters perception.

Suppose, for example, that we grew up with a myth showing pain as a sign of divine favor. Our perceptions and responses would be quite different: What looks like punishment to many might instead be welcome.

Do Spartan personalities "feel" pain? Presumably they do, since the Spartan personality has a body equipped with all the necessary nerve fibers and with a cerebral cortex and the brain cells that serve as a memory bank. But their worlds, their myths, and their personal histories enable them to deny the intruder access.

The conditions under which we perceive pain make a difference in what we feel. The most famous study of this part of the problem was made by Dr. H. K. Beecher, who found that infantrymen wounded on Anzio Beach during World War II demanded very little morphine for their pain. In fact, they demanded significantly less pain relief than did civilian patients suffering similar wounds or injuries. Beecher concluded that the wounded infantrymen saw their injuries as a decent way to get out of the greater pain of battle. A wound serious enough to send you back home was, if not entirely welcome in and of itself, at least better than a greater kind of agony and certainly better than death. Not so for the civilian. The wound suffered by a civilian doesn't send him anywhere, at least nowhere he wants to go. An injury or wound gets the infantryman out of a psychological mess; it puts other people into one.

Also, the brain can take only just so many signals at one time. I have already referred to the fact that active teaching, which calls for total concentration, pushed the pain in my hand into the background. I had much the same experience in hypnosis and self-hypnosis. Total concentration, then, on something outside the place that hurts will help to block out perception of pain, or at least alter it, even if only temporarily. Perhaps the Spartan personality can get his or her brain so busy with other matters that pain becomes relatively unimportant and therefore manageable. At least one pain theory helps to explain the neurological basis for this blocking activity, as we shall see.

Another minor point: Some pain persons find analgesic drugs unpleasant, especially those drugs strong enough to deal with severe pain. To these people the side effects seem just as bad as, if not worse than, "jabbing," "crushing," or "burning." Codeine gives you constipation. Morphine addles the mind. Percodan contains caffeine. So, pain persons who shove the drugs away are perhaps showing a little Spartan talent.

On the other hand, denying pain cannot be termed the ultimate in good things. It can in fact be a poor thing, when the pain being denied is of the short-term, acute variety. Nothing is gained by denying a belly ache, should it happen that a hot appendix is the stimulus. Anyway, Spartan types who might benefit from appropriate medical, surgical, or psychiatric help probably might as well make use of it and save their abilities for longer battles.

There is another, more ominous, side to denial. A pain person who denies the existence of his or her pain may simply be running away from reality. Facing the fact that the pain may well be untreatable may be so shattering that the person cannot admit its existence. Unfortunately, some pain persons can go on denying pain for months. And then, when the bad news finally gets through, they go to pieces. Not the best of experiences.

Anger
Anger, an emotion normally placed fairly low on the totem pole by experts in manners, religion, and self-control, is an-

other marker. If we have been led to believe that anger is bad form, or a sin, or self-indulgent behavior, then our predicament as pain persons becomes the more distressing. "Don't say those terrible things to the nice doctor!" "Don't scream!" "Don't hit the nurse!"

It matters very little what the experts in morality think. Anger is part of the pain way of life. Trying to insist that it isn't, or shouldn't be, is somewhat like saying that money problems don't or shouldn't affect a poor person's life. Nonsense. This failure of the imagination on the part of outsiders, with regard to the place of anger in the pain person's experience, leads to ugly consequences, like guilt and shame—the last things a pain person needs.

Anger, like the intruder that evokes it, presents itself in many different disguises: sometimes explosions of a fairly violent nature; often, just plain bitchiness; still more often, a constant state of jaundiced bitterness. (From an interview: "Did you throw things? I did. I would pick up a plate and throw it against the wall. . . . Well, no, I guess you couldn't do that, because of your hand. But I screamed and I threw things. Mostly, though, I was just crabby to everybody.") Perhaps bystanders can endure explosions, which don't last long, better than they can the ongoing Chinese water torture of endless small complaints. But both belong to the same general category.

Whatever causes individual expressions of anger belongs to the psyche, to the pain person's history. If we were taught to suppress anger, it may be that pain will produce less noise, a gentler bitchiness. If we grew up in a family of hot tempers, perhaps pain will produce broken dishes. In any case, the experience of pain produces startling transformations. Pain doesn't exactly bring out the "worst" in people; but it certainly provokes them. And if anger sometimes dismays the "innocent" bystander, it also dismays the pain person. ("I couldn't believe what I was saying to the doctor. I've never talked like that in my life. I just stood there and screamed, 'You have to do something.' Except I used some foul language.")

Anger, then, makes for interesting reactions, some of them quite unexpected. Pity that poor doctor. He's trying to do his best, and his patient is screaming at him. His medical education may have prepared him theoretically for this kind of encounter; but he too has emotions. Nobody can be educated for or inoculated against a head-on collision with an angry pain person. Also pity any pain person's family and friends. How embarrassing it all is! Why can't So-and-so behave more normally?

As in the case of denial, there are helpful and harmful aspects to the anger that accompanies the pain way. One obvious good effect is that anger has a certain therapeutic value; it engages us in action, if only the relatively feeble gesture of plate-smashing. Anger, being a by-product of fear, which itself gets lots of adrenalin bustling about the body, makes us want to do something, and I suspect that anything that makes the pain person want to do something can't be *all* bad. I'm speaking now, of course, about anger that is outwardly expressed. Sullen bitterness has little to recommend it. Nor, for that matter, does anger that turns inward, directing itself not to the intruder but to the self. Outwardly expressed, anger releases some of the emotional hurt that accompanies persistent pain. It purges.

The bad effects of anger are obvious. Pain persons who have no way of determining who the real enemy is may misdirect their anger, toward themselves sometimes, but more commonly toward others. The handiest objects, wives, husbands, parents, friends, have usually nothing at all to do with the origins of pain, save in the case of psychogenic pain. That is, although they affect perceptions and responses, they usually had nothing to do with the stimulus. Some very unpleasant side-effects will inevitably follow when the pain person's anger is directed toward those close to him or her. If anger is to do its best work, it should be directed at the intruder. How can one be angry at an abstract word or at an experience? Well, that is precisely what pain persons *are* angry at. Misplacing the emotion, failing to make use of it, further isolates the pain person from the reality of his or her experience.

Other bad effects result when the pain person directs the anger toward his or her doctor or toward the medical profession in general. We all ought to know by now that Dr. Kildare is not omnipotent. True, there are some bad doctors. But good doctors make mistakes, just as do mechanics, plumbers, computer programmers, and presidents. Yet when we get angry at what we think is poor service from them, our anger isn't usually taken to court. And if it is, the monetary rewards are usually minimal. When our anger takes a doctor to court, much more is at stake, including the cost of health insurance. (From a doctor: "Sure, the possibility of a malpractice suit makes a doctor move very cautiously [in treating pain]. He's not going to take risks.") Too bad so much anger-in-pain gets to court, especially since it ought to be obvious that an M.D. degree does not convey with it infallibility. Perhaps the average pain person could get relief faster if doctors weren't hobbled as they are. A much safer place toward which to direct all that angry energy would be something like the Social Security Administration or the welfare department or the people at Workman's Compensation. Bureaucracies don't mind being called names. They're used to it. Besides, there's nothing like a good fight with an agency to distract a pain person.

Depression

The unvarnished word "depression" never quite adequately describes what goes on in the pain person's psyche. For myself, I almost prefer to use "despair," since the two words have slightly different connotations. "Despair" means "without hope," which is where many pain persons are. That's the emotion conjured up by the information that there's no end in sight. "Depression" is a clinical word. When used in medical literature, it has certain defined meanings. Trained observers can spot it, while those who are untrained may not be able to see it at all, and those who are depressed may not know what ails them. It is, however, very nearly as devastating in its end results as any serious physical disease.

It, too, comes in assorted shapes, colors, and sizes. A depressed person can be angry, jittery, weepy, sullen, passive, active, agitated, and/or docile. Everything depends on what's inside the big circle in the diagram. There are levels of depression, too. It ranges from mild to severe.

Painful as depression is, some people (including many who are not traveling the pain way) prefer to deny that they're in it. We do admit to feeling depressed when it's a short-term thing, as when the "wrong" team wins the Superbowl or when a Christmas present fails to please. When external events make us feel blue, we will feel fine as soon as they clear up. But the more serious forms of depression come from the inside; changes in the external world have little or no effect.

Why do we deny depression? We fear it, and we fear letting others see the intensity of our emotions. "Depressed? Who, me? Don't be ridiculous." Still, the symptoms are unmistakable: changes in sleeping and eating habits; loss of interest in work and sex; withdrawal from the arena of human relationships; inability to laugh. Anyone who has ever dealt with a pain person will recognize the symptoms. Unfortunately, denial of depression is something like denial of a broken leg. Denial ultimately costs much more time, money, and energy than medical care. And, since the chronic pain person will almost inevitably experience some degree of depression, he or she had better prepare to deal with it.

Although it seems unlikely, depression does afford one golden opportunity, providing, of course, that the pain person admits its existence. It can elicit a call for help. It did in my case. Depression is like sitting in a pool of tears. When it dawns on us that we are getting wet and that it's cold outside, we can yell for someone to give us a hand up. And, once standing, we can begin to move again. Being in motion is much more comfortable than sitting in a pool.

Another "good" effect has two sides to it. Depression gets us all some gains in sympathy and attention, as everyone races nervously about, trying to get us to smile. As we already know, however, excess sympathy makes the pain person's plight worse. Yet sympathy offered on the basis of realistic understanding of depression's dangers does help. And when the trained observer notes depression, help will be forthcoming.

The bad effects of depression need not be restated. Withdrawal from love and laughter, from people around us, from the big wide world, compounds the pain person's difficulties. Now that I remember Mr. A, stuck in the hypothetical snail shell I imagined for him, I would have to say that he's depressed as well as angry. Someone really should reach him, get him up and moving along the way again, because he may be killing himself. To be sure, not every case of severe depression leads to suicide, but some do. As a British doctor observed, suicides are the tip of the depression iceberg. They are visible. What we need to identify is the other 9/10ths of the iceberg, the part submerged.

Acceptance

Acceptance happens to be a slippery word. It has a passive quality about it, a sort of "You can't fight City Hall, so why bother?" connotation. In this sense, "acceptance" comes to mean "surrender," giving in, giving up, lying down and (for all practical purposes) dying. If pain persons move toward that kind of acceptance, they gradually turn into passive prisoners of the intruder, thereby damaging not only themselves but other pain persons. As a mileage marker, indeed, "surrender" signals the end of the road.

Acceptance-as-surrender carries other dangers with it. Once the pain person has given up, he or she has so adapted to the terms of surrender that no other way of life seems possible or even desirable. To use the prisoner of war analogy, once we have adjusted to life in a POW camp and have resigned ourselves to its discomforts, we might even resist efforts to set us free. Thus do many pain persons become professional prisoners, even to the extent of enjoying the fact that they baffle the doctors and outwit the experts, all of which does no good to anyone. What percentage of pain persons get themselves sucked into the acceptance-as-surrender trap, I don't know. I do know it is a tempting trap.

When I learned that my hands would never be restored to their original condition, that my thumbs and wrists would never function "normally," I took a brief look at the "prisoner" trap. Handicapped for life. Well, why not stay on permanent Total Disability, why not collect from my pension fund and from Social Security? Why not stay where I am, now that the neurostimulators at least take care of the worst pain? For some reason I still don't understand, the options did not attract me for very long. But I remember the temptation.

Acceptance can mean something else, however. It can go far beyond surrender and develop into hard-nosed fact facing, including understanding of the situation, emotional and mental assessment of the consequences of pain, and a brand-new way of life.

All pain persons can take lessons in this sort of acceptance from paraplegics and quadraplegics. Whatever the reasons they find themselves in their wheelchairs, they usually develop remarkable ability to face facts. True, they probably can no longer cavort up and down stairs; true, they have to accommodate themselves to a lot of unpleasantness; true, a lot of what most people consider "life" has shut its doors; and true, some jobs are out of the question. But realistic acceptance provides them with what outsiders cannot quite understand: an altered view of what to the rest of us looks like a dead end. Similar acceptance gives a new perspective to the experience of persistent pain. (From an interview: "I hate it now when people offer to do things for me. I have to try. I told my husband not to baby me, but sometimes he still does. When I need his help, I ask for it. Otherwise, he's supposed to let me fend for myself, even when the pain is pretty bad.")

Acceptance-as-response, then, is nothing like acceptance-as-surrender. As a mileage marker, it is not the final one. It points pain persons in new directions. Or, to return to the terminology of war, it develops into a technique for planning a breakout from the POW camp.

It is critically important for a pain person and everyone around one to understand where he or she is, within this way of life. Angry depressed people ought not to be treated as if they should have been raised to be Spartans, for instance. Nor should passive prisoners be treated as if they were free. It is also critically important to keep in mind at all times that nothing is constant in the pain experience. Even if it could be staked out, or pinned down like a butterfly, it belongs to a living, breathing, human organism, which brings us to a very lofty dimension of the problem—that of philosophy.

It used to be that philosophers dealt in terms of mind (or soul) and body. They reasoned mightily within those terms. When they talked about pain, then, they talked about it as a "thing" belonging exclusively to one realm or the other, thus inducing a lot of unhelpful experiments and producing a lot of irrelevant graphs and articles. To this day, a good many researchers still operate from what must be termed a 17th century "mind-body" dualism. Newer schools of thought about pain rely on existentialism. But the most useful philosophy of pain emerges from the work of Alfred North Whitehead, the mathematician-philosopher.

Whitehead, like Einstein, had the genius to perceive that *time,* like length or breadth, is a dimension of the physical universe. He also had the genius to perceive that the observer of an experiment (and this applies to those who conduct experiments designed to measure pain) is *part of the experiment.* One cannot detach the clinician from the 28 healthy American college students' reactions to painful stimuli administered in laboratories. When it comes down to the laws of physics, just as our bodies are made up of constantly moving particles or electrical charges (atoms), so our experiences of pain are made up of moving parts and shifting qualities. There's no avoiding it: The problem of pain does not sit still for those of us who would like to get a permanent handle on it. If it did, we might manage to find its final solution. But the problem, like those who endure it, is always changing. So the final dimension is one of mobility. Pain persons, although they rarely know it, are always changing. They *are* mobile, although they don't think so. They desperately need to know their own state.

One more thing needs saying. No long-term pain person can ever "go home" again, "home" being the way things used to be, that environment of facts and possibilities, the multitude of emotions, relationships, and self-images which used to be taken for granted. The intruder's invasion changed everything.

For one thing, pain cripples. A bricklayer afflicted with LBP can no longer work as a bricklayer; he has to find another way. A teacher can no longer carry a full teaching load; an executive can no longer sit at his desk for ten hours or have two martinis before lunch (alcohol and potent painkillers do not mix happily); a secretary can no longer type; a young mother can no longer lift her toddler; a student can no longer attend classes; and so on, *ad infinitum*. Pain persons and those who minister to them have to learn that there is no way back, no retreat to safety.

But not being able to go "home" again need not prove fatal, even if the pain persists for a lifetime. Everything depends on who's in charge of the operation:

> As the diversity, and undefined limits, of all the circumstances bring a great number of factors into consideration in War, as the most of these factors can only be estimated according to probability, therefore, if the Chief of an Army does not bring to bear upon them a mind with an intuitive perception of the truth, a confusion of ideas and views must take place, in the midst of which the judgment will become bewildered.
> —*von Clausewitz*

4

Strategy,
or How Do We Cope?

Developing a strategy, or master battle plan, requires more than casual guessing games and clinical findings; as von Clausewitz pointed out, the Chief of an Army who does not know what he's doing will surely fail. Discovering the dimensions of the pain situation is, of course, the first step. No general worth his pay would dream of embarking on the development of a strategy unless he knew not only the objectives to be accomplished, but the political angles to be considered, his own strengths and weaknesses, and the strengths and weaknesses of his enemy.

In the ways of the world, generals have an easier time than pain persons. The average pain person, faced with the shattering news that he or she can not "go home" again, usually has no idea at all what the dimensions of the pain problem are. He or she has an immediate objective, to be sure: to kill or immobilize the intruder. Unfortunately if the pain is persistent, that objective may not be attainable, a fact that nearly everybody would like to ignore. Generals are trained for this sort of impasse. Pain persons aren't. Generals can alter objectives. Pain persons can't, or think they can't.

Again, generals can appreciate the political aspects of war and can take them into account when planning ahead. Pain persons are usually totally unaware of the ripple effects created by their experience and by their responses to pain. They continue, at their own risk, to believe that pain belongs to them individually. Having lost touch with the world, sensing themselves to be besieged, they don't notice that their pain, although isolating them from "normal" people, has profound effect on those who live around them.

When it comes to assessing strengths and weaknesses, the military have all kinds of advantages. Generals can count troops and weapons, can allocate their money to aircraft, artillery, infantry, paratroops, and so forth, as they draw up their plans. They can cover soft spots in their defenses, knowing ahead of time what the soft spots are. Pain persons, on the other hand, are usually quite helpless in making assessments. The intruder has a nasty habit of demolishing what were once thought to be personal strengths and of attacking precisely the most vulnerable places, particularly in the psyche.

As to knowledge about the enemy, once more the military have an advantage; they have ways and means of gathering intelligence, of counting the enemies' troops and weapons, of spotting an incipient invasion, of sifting and weighing evidence. Doctors probably count as intelligence gatherers in the pain process. But, unfortunately, they do not always agree as to how to treat the evidence they gather. Pain persons have to do most of their own intelligence work, and for the most part, they haven't the foggiest idea where to start. Ronald Melzack was accurate in entitling his book *The Puzzle of Pain*. A puzzle it is. Yet no strategy—in war or in pain

—can accomplish much, without some understanding of the intruder, without determining the puzzle's rules.

In sum, the individual pain person is usually woefully underequipped and undertrained for the battle he or she has to direct.

And, for better or worse, like it or not, it *is* the individual who must direct the battle, must be in charge of the pain experience. Doctors cannot draw up the plans; they can help, of course, by supplying needed information, and other people can help, by being observers or by offering tactical support. But no one can do for a pain person what he or she must do. Somebody has to be in charge; somebody has to take responsibility. In war, it's up to the generals; in pain, it's up to the pain person. All too often, pain persons try to turn the whole process over to the medical profession, in the quite mistaken assumption that the doctors are in charge. When they do so, they unwittingly resign from the fight, frequently with poor results, like a military commander who turns over his command to a subordinate and expects not to have to make any plans at all.

Pain persons rarely know that they can fight back, nor do they understand that those who fight back stand the best chance of living fruitfully within the pain way of life. One pain person of my acquaintance is a real fighter. As it happens, she competed in several sports before she got damaged. After an initial period of passive depression, her competitive instincts came back into play and are now proving invaluable. She deals with her present situation realistically, whereas another kind of personality might have curled up in a shell like Mr. A.

All this ignorance about the pain experience is quite understandable, if not quite forgiveable, especially among doctors. Coping with persistent pain frequently seems to be a full time job, although it needn't be. And few people with full time jobs have anything to spare for education. A better view would be one which presents pain education as on-the-job training. In assembling this book, for instance, I learned a great deal about pain in general; I also learned, on the side, a great deal about my own brand of it.

As has already been noted, the development of a strategy also requires conscious awareness of the individuality of the pain experience. Bluntly speaking, there can be no single universal plan, for doctors or for pain persons; each plan must be tailor-made, which is perhaps the reason for many failures in treatment. (No one form of pain control works for everyone. The percentage of failure is surprisingly high.) For pain persons to rely on medical breakthroughs is foolish; they have to make their own breakthroughs.

The first logical step in strategy-building is that of erasure. Erasure means wiping away. You can't draw a diagram on a blackboard, the way military men do, when the blackboard is all covered up with useless speculations that serve no purpose and may indeed be far out of date, if not totally inappropriate. Some marks on a blackboard can be wiped off with a brush of the finger; some need to be erased with a patented dust-free chalk remover; some will go away only with soap and water. A few have to fade away with exposure to air and sunlight. As the blackboard gets cleaned, the pain person can begin to sketch his or her own position and thus form a tentative plan.

What kinds of things should be categorized as "useless speculations"? Well, one kind begins with that notoriously unhelpful phrase "if only." "If only" never solved anything, so far as I can tell. And where pain is concerned, it's a drag, a hindrance. "If only the doctor would operate," for instance: The doctor either will or will not. "If only" has little bearing on the decision. In fact, "if only," under some conditions involving surgery, can be terribly destructive. A pain person may plead for surgery, a surgeon may give in and operate, and the operation may make matters worse. Persons suffering psychogenic pain may get multiple surgical treatments; but surgery cannot touch a lesion that doesn't exist. Result? An unhappy, resentful pain person and a frustrated surgeon. In the meanwhile, of course, the intruder keeps right on tunneling away, even beneath the defense perimeters of psychogenic pain persons.

Or, "if only" I had been more careful with that back-hoe, with the car, with the sail. Backward looking "if only's" lead straight into blame and guilt, which are not the best frames of mind within which to plan strategically. The true dimensions of the problem of pain may well include events and processes that might have gone some other way, and someone may have been at fault; but on the whole it is wiser to admit retrospective anger and not to let it curdle into wishful thinking. The assault of pain cannot be altered, even if it is now only a memory. It happened. No "if only" ever invented can change the past.

Then there's the "if only" that creates havoc among those around the pain person, the very people needed as supporting troops. "If only people realized what hell this is!" "If only Marge or Jack or Tony or the boss understood what it's like!" They don't, and they probably never will. Even if one of them were attacked by the same intruder and wound up with the same kind of persistent pain, they still wouldn't understand exactly. As we have seen, the sense of community in pain is severely limited. This particular "if only" derives from a self-centered assumption that all pain persons are alike, whereas each pain person has a different story to tell. Pretending there are no differences clouds the issue of strategy-building and further complicates the possibility of finding out what pain persons *do* have in common.

"If only" the pain would go away. Maybe it will, and maybe it won't. Whether it does or not has nothing to do with "if only."

Then there are others: a new pain pill, which isn't addictive, which really works, which doesn't cost much, which doesn't have nasty side effects; a new surgical technique that is guaranteed to work; a change of climate; a new invention; a fat inheritance from a hitherto unknown benefactor, which will take care of the bills (in and of themselves a secondary pain). These "if only's" and others get us precisely nowhere. Worse still, they inhibit our ability to face reality. They have their own insidious allure—all daydreams do. Unlike ordinary daydreams, however, which can produce workable ideas, "if only" thinking paralyzes the pain person.

Once "if only" is expunged, another slogan can be chalked up in its place. This one reads: *"Now that."*

Some of the myths at least have to be examined and insofar as possible erased. Myths probably cannot be entirely wiped out, because they are so buried that half the time we don't even know they are there, and because they may still have some degree of validity. We all grew up knowing them unconsciously, much as we know that black cats are peculiar, that red sunsets promise fair weather, and that "good fences make good neighbors." We can't get at myths with soap and water. About the best we can do is to dig out the ones we can find and let fresh air and sunshine gradually fade their influence.

One of the worst examples of the unconscious power of a myth can be observed in the clinical evidence that many chronic pain persons were, as children, treated to pain experiences too heavy for them to manage: child abuse. A healthy percentage of child abuse victims turn up later on as adult pain persons. For these people, pain very early became a bizarre substitute for affection and attention. After all, if the only notice a child is given by mother or father happens to be a beating, whipping, burning, or worse, then the experience of pain will equal "attention." It will certainly be assumed to be *punishment,* and it will certainly have overtones of *expiation,* since the child-abusing parent probably is making the child a scapegoat for his or her own psychic pain. Perhaps this myth area truly belongs to the psychiatrists and social workers. Yet professional helpers cannot do their jobs until the adult pain person who is dragging the myths around is ready to have them brought to light. No pain strategy can be mapped out until they are.

The myths are hard to abandon. They closely resemble moral and ethical codes. But once they are exposed, and we see them for what they are, some of their power may be dissipated.

What else needs erasing? It would be helpful if we could take our patented dust-free chalk remover to the world around us and remove all the misconceptions about pain that so heavily burden persons struggling along its way. It would be helpful; but it probably is not possible. For example, no matter how often we are told that "psychogenic" pain and "hypochondriac" pain are *real,* that they exist, that they hurt, somewhere somebody is going to be saying, in arrogant ignorance, "It's all in the head." Yes, indeed, and so is organic pain. I suppose the best that can be accomplished is that pain persons learn not to feel guilty about the implied accusations. Psychogenic pain is a complex event. It may have begun with an injury, a measurable "organic" wound. Over the years, however, and despite successful treatment of the wound, the pain may have continuted unabated. Doctors can find nothing more to do, while the pain person continues to complain. The doctors put "psychogenic" on the chart, and that seems to be that—except that the pain persists. A habit of perception and response has developed, and because it has, there's no need for anyone to go into a decline. And there certainly is no call for anyone in perfect health to comment. Of course, no single person can alter the way the world thinks about such terms as "psychogenic" and "hypochondriac" and "psychosomatic." But anyone, especially someone who is ignorant of such matters, can learn to understand that the connotations of the words are nothing more than connotations—nasty, free-floating associations, with little scientific significance.* I have yet to meet anyone who hasn't, at one time or another, suffered from one or another of these kinds of pain.

Other things need to be erased. For one, the notion (where it comes from I cannot imagine) that there are victories and defeats of some cosmic nature in the battle of pain. Since pain is a process, it is questionable whether unconditional victory is possible. Military history teaches otherwise: World War I led inevitably to World War II, via what we all naively thought was victory. World War II led to the Cold War, and "unconditional surrender" was merely a step along the way. There was no final victory or final defeat in Korea or in Vietnam, no matter who's doing the talking. There were, however, a lot of casualties.

---

*The three words, it must be emphasized, *do* have their place in the vocabulary of medicine, which is where they belong. I am here talking about common, everyday usage.

So it is with pain, especially what is called "intractable" pain, the kind for which doctors have no cure. Pain persons have deliberately to expel from their minds the marketplace hunger for finality; and victory and defeat, as concepts, have to be modified to suit special circumstances, if they are to be anything but disappointments. Our human itch to make everything turn out "right," to find bad (pain) and good (absence of pain) dealt out according to some rule book, blocks the way. Human beings love simple solutions. Unhappily, in the pain way of life there are none. No final victory. No final defeat. Each onslaught has to be faced as it comes, with the firm understanding that it is only a skirmish, a small win or loss, not a final state, for the only final state is death.

So much for erasure, although each pain person may have to decide what other platitudes and useless speculations need to be washed away.

How do we go about constructing a strategy, once we have some space in which to compose it?

Here it might be wise to emphasize again that only the pain person can develop the right strategy. If we look back at the last diagram in Part III, it will be apparent that no two pain individuals have precisely the same internal materials with which to work. Presumably we have by now, once and for all, discarded as useless the notion that pain is a thing; now we know it to be an impediment. In terms of long-range planning, that notion diminishes flexibility, and war requires flexibility. So does the battle against pain. The enemy, in both cases, is neither a fortress nor a stone wall, waiting around to be demolished, whether by dynamite or an act of God. In other words, pain, like Attila the Hun or the Nazis, doesn't lie down and wait for things to happen. It moves around, attacks in unexpected ways, probes and searches for vulnerable spots. Hence the need to develop a strategy that allows for tactical changes, for shifting circumstances, for alterations in the situation and problem.

As must surely be obvious by now, the first strategic step is the tough-minded acceptance of pain as a way of life—no cheating allowed. Such a level cannot be reached, for instance, if there are "if only's" hanging around the edges. If the doctors say there is nothing they can do, or that they have done all they can, it is probably reasonable to check around for a second or third opinion. But there comes a time when shopping around becomes unrewarding and very expensive. I can remember asking three doctors, sequentially, whether my hands would ever get well, whether the nerves would regenerate themselves (nerves sometimes do). The first doctor said no. So I asked the second doctor, and he said no. So I asked the third doctor, and he said no. I could have saved my breath; but I was unwilling to accept the chilling implications of what they said. When I finally did, acceptance brought relief. For just so long as I was wistfully hoping that things could be as they once were, I was keeping myself from doing what I should have been doing—that is, working out a way to live with a partial handicap.

Acceptance of the fact of persistent pain can hardly be called the easiest of human tasks. It never quite seems fair that some people are singled out to travel that way. And oh, what damage that fiction of "fairness" manufactures for pain persons! Whoever said that the world (or God) was "fair"? Once we admit that goodness does not always triumph, that moral purity does not guarantee freedom from suffering, acceptance becomes much easier.

And once we achieve some measure of acceptance, other things, nice things, start happening. For one thing, priorities can be rearranged, an important step in formulating strategy.

Of what everlasting importance is one's golf score? Will any one of us make the Guinness Book of Records for consecutive days of prayer for relief of pain? How many parcels do we have to carry to win whatever we're trying to win? What are the pain person's priorities? Can they be left in their present order, or ought they to be reshuffled and some discarded?

Acceptance, then, brings with it the curiously comforting opportunity to sort out what matters and what doesn't. The pain person may be astonished at how much can be tossed out as not worth the effort. In this sense, the religious conviction that pain purifies the soul turns out to be remarkably apt. Pain does purify, in that it strips away our illusions. Once upon a time, I thought that my piano was an essential part of my life. When I could no longer play it without making so many mistakes that I couldn't stand the sound of my own music, I did a lot of weeping. Then it dawned on me that I never did play with more than amateur style, even at my best. I still have the piano, and it looks very nice in the living room. But I have no regrets. One illusion stripped away, one priority put where it always belonged, somewhere at the bottom of the list.

Acceptance of the pain way includes living in a world that was never designed for pain persons. It does not include running away and hiding. Pain persons have to adjust themselves to the world, because, as they will certainly discover, the world is not going to change for anyone or for all of us. For example, nobody wants to hear the pain-full story, just as nobody wants to hear about someone else's bankruptcy proceedings. Acceptance seems to bring with it diminishment of the urge to "show and tell." The story becomes boring not just to those who listen, but to those who are talking. Again, consider riding in a car. It may no longer be possible to sit in one position for more than an hour or two, let alone drive. Lots of people, pain persons and others, have found out that it *is* possible to stop a car, to get out, and to walk around. Acceptance of the limitations imposed by the intruder creates its own benefits: Pain persons who must get out of the car, and walk around, see the landscape that used to go by so fast that it might as well not have existed.

Which brings to light the fascinating truth that acceptance of pain uncovers a great deal about the world in which we all live. Pain persons can see things that others cannot. The best definition of acceptance, that is, clear-headed facing up to the demands and rewards of the way things really are, has promises within it, not simply penalties.

The second phase of strategy development is that of opening the eyes and the ears. This phase is painful, in and of itself, because it entails finding out a lot of facts about ourselves, whether we be pain persons, doctors, families, or friends. A pain person needs to come to know his or her own stake in the life of pain; so must those around him or her. To appreciate the magnitude of that stake requires careful visualizing and hearing. Perhaps the pain person does have some Spartan talents; and perhaps, owing to past hurts and past events associated with pain, those talents got covered up or overlooked. They're probably still there, waiting to be exercized. Those talents are like poker chips. They can be used; but they cannot be used until they have been brought into play. And they cannot be brought into play until they have been identified.

Eye and ear opening takes some will power and considerable effort at insight into the pain problem, as well as a sense of adventure; and I suppose these demands account for the fact that many pain persons resist help and grimly hang on to their pain. It isn't that they actually enjoy the spot they're in: depending on others, confounding the physicians, using up time and money. On the contrary, they are probably afraid to take the first step out. Do I enjoy my painful state? That's a tough question, because it demands an answer based on inner honesty, and honesty may have been warped by the intruder's assault. For my part, I think that most pain persons *do* enjoy their experience, if only a bit. It does gain attention. It does attract sympathy. Of course, no one enjoys severe attacks; but persistent pain is what the experts describe as "benign." If it weren't benign, body tissues would be undergoing destruction (as in cancer) and there would be nothing left to hurt. In its benign (strange word for pain) moments, then, the pain way of life can not only be endured, but may be secretly enjoyed. The issue of enjoyment needs to be raised, because only by responding to it openly can the pain person become aware of the temptations discussed in Part III.

Opened eyes and ears also afford access to some interesting facts about behavior, that of pain persons, doctors, families, and friends. For outsiders, seeing and listening to what goes on in the pain person's life means paying close attention to something other than surface signals: Grandma's whining and complaining may or may not be necessary. Everyone around her knows her complaints are irritating, but perhaps they indicate something to which attention should be paid. On the other hand, the pain person, the insider, may discover some interesting facts about himself or herself, and with opened eyes and ears, may even develop keen sensibilities about the pain way. Pain persons must be treated correctly, and correct treatment demands accurate vision and hearing; it also requires that the pain person see and hear accurately.

Doctors are not without fault in this area. Pain persons are not every doctor's favorite kind of patient. A neurosurgeon informs me that doctors get secondary gains from treating some patients, much as pain persons get secondary gains from their pain (attention and sympathy). Doctors look for the satisfaction of cures and of treating interesting lesions. When they don't get secondary gains, they are likely to wish to refer the patient on to someone else—"referred" pain. The same neurosurgeon, in answer to a question having to do with what he found most helpful in the treatment of pain, said, "Communication." He then went on to explain that "Communication includes honesty, language, trust, and concern." He said that he could not treat dishonest patients.

His definition of communication is interesting, because it suggests that the pain person's own character or personality has as much to do, if not more, with the surgeon's success as does skill with a scalpel. Dull, uninvolved patients rarely respond; insightful patients do better. In other words, the hangers-on already identified are poor prospects for relief; the passive POW is not a good candidate for surgical treatment of pain; dishonest patients are only camp followers. "Concern" is a term that works in two directions: The doctor must be concerned about the patient, naturally; but the patient must be concerned about himself or herself and about helping the doctor. There's little to be gained from surgery for pain if the patient tells lies about levels and degrees; if he or she refuses to talk (just writhes and moans); if he or she mistrusts the medical profession to such an extent that failure is anticipated before the anesthesiologist gets started; or if the patient is so inwardly turned as not to care about anything.*

---

*The influence of character and personality on the pain experience is documented by clinical findings with reference to post-operative pain. The kind and degree of fear shown by the patient before surgery has a great deal to do with the kind and

Perhaps the greatest advantage to be gained from opened eyes and ears is that of education. The seeing and hearing pain person has the opportunity to acquire the education for living with pain that successful military personnel get for their careers. But in all education, including grammar schools and colleges, the student has to do most of the work. The student puts it all together. So it is with pain education. Open eyes and ears allow for communication among all those concerned. But no good will come of it, unless the pain person makes use of that which is being communicated.

The third phase of strategy-building is somewhat more concrete. This is the development of personal goals. Pain persons usually say that their primary goal is to get rid of pain. But such is not always the case, and in any event, sometimes pain cannot be eliminated. Pain persons also frequently say, staring fixedly at the "Let's all go home again" mirage, that their goal is to resume work or housework or snowmobiling or what-have-you. They may not be able to do so.

If a pain person can't go home again, where does he or she go? If the obvious goals are phantoms, how does he or she direct all the energy stored up to be used for goal-making and tending?

Adopting the idea of moving somewhere else, grasping that idea firmly and steadily, is like making the first stroke in a strategic diagram. If an army cannot move north, it will have to move north-northeast, or even westward. The necessity to move in a different direction sets everyone's mind to work on "possibilities," one of the finest words in the English language for pain persons. Within the pain process, there are

---

degree of pain suffered afterward. Character and personality are contained within the diagrams, specifically within the small circle "History."

so many personal variables lying around, waiting to be noticed and tested, that every pain individual has the opportunity to start a new life, one that includes pain, to be sure, but one that proves exciting because it is new. Once the pain person begins to think about what is possible, it takes only a pinch of imagination to start constructing a new "home," new goals.

The pain clinics (more about them later) report great success in helping pain persons to construct new lives for themselves. Once out of bed (as it were) and moving about, being praised and encouraged for each accomplishment, pain persons apparently change their self-images. They stop looking at themselves as helpless, hopeless cripples and learn to value their own skills and abilities. When they go "home," it may be to the same house or apartment, but it's a new "home" because they are different people. All this despite persistent pain and usually with little medication.

Similar turnarounds take place outside pain clinics. Psychotherapy can be enormously helpful in the goal-setting area. (And in case anyone is fretting about the cost of psychotherapy, it needn't last for ten years and it needn't cost excessively. Community mental health centers, which are inexpensive, are more numerous than one might think.) Psychotherapy helps the pain person uncover the potentially useful variables and bring forward buried talents and interests. People with Lower Back Pain may no longer be able to work a back-hoe or shuffle files around or hoist sails; they can do other things. They can still work with their hands, talk to people, think, do arithmetic, teach, and, most important, help other pain people with *their* battles.

Sometimes the turnaround seems a sudden, unthought-out decision: "I'm not going to live like this any longer." Pain persons have been known to make spur of the moment choices, as if impelled to remake their lives. One person might decide to go to night school to finish off a high school education, or to take courses at a community college with a view to getting into a new line of work. Another might suddenly decide to apply for vocational rehabilitation and counseling. Another might decide that volunteer work (there's a lot of it waiting to be done) is better than no work at all, and definitely better than sitting or lying around the house all day. Still another might choose a hobby suitable for physical and emotional needs. Such individual efforts cannot always be made without outside help, but the decision-making moment represents one more indication of the fact that pain persons have to map their own strategies. Before they can do so, they must wish to do so.

It should also be noted, however, that the setting of goals, the making of a new "home," has to include a healthy component of reality. Some goals, however interesting and attractive, will probably be unattainable, and I can see little sense in encouraging an LBP to take violin lessons if there's no interest in music among the variables. Over against what the pain person would like to be able to do must be set what he or she is able to do. It took me a year and a half to figure out that full-time teaching was far too exhausting and far too costly (in terms of damage to my hands) to be a realistic goal. So I had to opt for part-time teaching instead. Also, the goals set by pain persons have to be flexible enough to allow for changes along the way. The way may take unexpected turns, as do the people in it.

One final warning. Pain persons setting new goals are probably going to be frightened. Generally speaking, it *is* safer, if you can stand it, to stay in place, even when "place" includes pain. When fright inhibits motion, outsiders can offer help, assuming that they know how and when to do so.

Encouragement, yes. Willingness to help, yes. And sensitivity to know when not to help. Outsiders can pose the difficult questions: So you want to change jobs; what about transportation? So you want to go back to school; can you sit at a desk for fifty minutes? So you want to set up a home workshop; can we afford the expense? With appropriate help, the vague threats contained in the formation of goals, threats which are really tactical in nature, are allayed in the excitement of planning.

Now we have started to see how strategies take shape.

First, strategy is the responsibility of the pain person, who must take charge of his or her own destiny.

Second, strategy is based on the understanding that pain is an ongoing process.

Third, strategy depends for its effectiveness on open communication and self-education.

Fourth, strategy is directed toward fresh, new goals.

Von Clausewitz said it best: "what is required of an officer is . . . knowledge . . . and good judgment." Everything depends on who's in charge. If no one is in charge, as is all too often the case with the pain way of life, hope gets lost in the shuffle, and the pain way becomes a never-ending nightmare.

Because the individual pain person is ultimately responsible for strategic planning, it is impossible to outline a universal, all-purpose model that would apply to each and every case. Most of the time, pain persons, like all other human beings, are unaware of what they are doing and why. Only 20/20 hindsight reveals the details of the planning process. So I have to reflect on my own experience to demonstrate how the development of strategy works out in real life.

Now that I can look back, not in anger but in surprise, I can see that I had a great deal of erasing to do. I carried around with me more idle speculations than was seemly. I used to dream about surgical procedures I had heard about: injection of alcohol into the nerve to kill it, for instance; even amputation (this before my left hand began to hurt, obviously). I had a bagful of "if only's," but the most seductive of all was the one about "if only people would understand." It wasn't until I began to notice that no one was all that interested that I began to realize that no one *could* understand. Then there was the backward glance "if only." Had I not gripped my ball-point pen the way I did, had I not been angry at some of my colleagues while I was gripping the pen, had I not insisted on writing out my lecture notes and class plans in longhand, and so on, maybe none of my hand problems would have happened. And, as would be expected, "if only" the pain would go away.

Erasing those speculations took quite a while—at least two years, as I recall. I don't remember making any conscious efforts to get rid of them, although I now wish I had had the sense to do so. Rather, they slowly faded away as time passed. Then again, I was lucky. Circumstances and people helped me shove them aside, inch by inch.

The myths I had to contend with were unearthed during psychotherapy. I had been most afflicted by the pain = punishment and pain = expiation ones. It took a lot of hard work to bring them to light. But once they were visible, they did in fact lose their grip on my imagination. God was *not* punishing me. I hadn't consciously thought He was, but deep down inside the myth was directing me without my knowledge. Similarly, the "expiation" myth turned out to have its basis in nothing more significant than some ill-digested childhood memories. Once exposed, that too lost its power.

Defusing the power of my myths took about a year, but it was time well spent.

Somewhere during this time of erasing, something curious happened. I began to look at myself with a little detachment, and I saw that my self-image had not been entirely accurate. I thought I had certain strengths and found that I had deceived myself. I turned out not to be the tough-minded, realistic person I had thought. On the contrary, I behaved impulsively and frequently acted on the basis of inadequate information, both in my job and with relation to my pain experience. I always insisted on doing as much as possible by myself. All things considered, that insistence was about as stupid a form of stubborness as I ever indulged in. I think it was when I dropped a heavy pot of onion soup that I decided there were some things I shouldn't be trying to do. In terms of the pain experience, sporadic and uncontrolled outbursts like mine are not helpful in the building of strategy. But they may indicate a source of energy that, properly guided, can prove useful.

I had always thought I could deal with doctors as a reasonable, intelligent, calm, cool person. What a joke that assumption turned out to be! I was irrational, foolish, jittery, and uncool. Once I developed an awareness of my weakness in the medical arena, things eased up. I learned to explain to doctors how much I feared them, and they in turn were better able to help me. On the other hand, what I had secretly thought a form of moral weakness—making jokes out of unlikely material—turned out to be a strength. I organized a course on "The Comic Perspective," and in so doing learned a lot about dealing with pain.*

---

*I learned, for instance, that the comic perspective demands detachment. We don't laugh when our dear grandfather slips on a banana peel, only when an anonymous authority figure does. Only when we move away from ugly things can we laugh at

The victory-defeat mode of thinking lasted only a short while. There were too many of each for me to think of a single one in final terms. Each time I thought the whole battle was over, something else happened, so that I became accustomed to the tenuousness of victories and defeats. Once I slipped and fell on an icy back porch. I grabbed for the railing, and, in so doing, pulled some internal wiring in my neurostimulator. I hadn't done any irreparable damage, but I had to wear my left arm in a sling for months. The immobilization of my forearm in turn caused another problem in my left hand, one that took two more months to correct. But by that time I had learned not to view a minor setback as a major defeat. I had also learned something that most pain persons have to learn—that is, not to panic at the prospect of a setback. If the pain way is a permanent or very long-term one, one can afford a setback now and then.

Acceptance of pain as a way of life was very difficult for me, because I had always believed in the "pain-as-thing" fallacy. It has taken me the better part of five years to reject surrender in favor of realism. Today, there may be small echoes of acceptance-as-surrender singing away in the back of my mind, but I have little time to listen to them. Once in a while I wonder if I'll ever be able to go back to Dr. X and say, "Okay, you can remove the neurostimulators; I'm over it." Then something happens—the barometer takes a nose dive or I overuse my hands—and I'm back on the way again. It's good exercise for my psyche. In terms of prognosis, I simply don't know what will happen tomorrow or next month or next year. Dr. X says, "Any time you say so, I'll take them out." When that will be, I don't know, and I *have* learned not to ask, because pushing for a target date called

them. The same thing might be said about pain. To cope with the pain experience, we need detachment.

"end of the way" would counteract acceptance. Meanwhile, I'm a pain person.

The fairness of it all—or, rather, the unfairness—bothered me very much. Why me? Intellectually, I knew that "fairness" is a concept derived from human ideals, from Utopian urges toward justice. I also knew the Book of Job, which is as good a dramatization of unfairness as ever crept into the history of human thought. Still, I had never cast myself in the role of Job, and it came as something of a shock to realize that the "patience" of Job means nothing more world-shattering than the "suffering" of Job. Only when I figured out (and that too took time) that the "me" I was groaning over was not the center of the universe, did I get out of the morass.

As to priorities and the need to re-organize them, that operation was relatively simple for me, although I realize it may be difficult for others. When you are fighting to stay in motion, to keep on *living* in the pain way, all sorts of clutter just naturally fall by the wayside. I have always loved to cook, still do; but now I use my gourmet cookbook for reading rather than for cooking, since my hands cannot do what is required for fancy cookery. I can't play the piano, but I no longer care. I can't carry more than about eight pounds of groceries, but I'm not ashamed to ask for help. I ask students to help me with my books, which is a good example of priority rearrangement: Which is more important? Being the "in charge," self-sufficient, aloof teacher, or being sensible about what my hands will take? Yes, pain does purify.

The opening of eyes and ears hurt a lot, almost more than my hands did. I did not enjoy being subjected to what I, at least, interpreted as attacks on my honesty, as when one of my colleagues rudely remarked, "Your hands can't be all that bad—you're still smoking cigarettes." I couldn't explain the neuroanatomy of the hand then, and I suspect he continues to believe that there's an element of hypochondria at work in me. He may be right, but it doesn't matter, really. I did, for a time, enjoy all the "oohs" and "ahs" and "how brave you are's." Consequently, I resented it when outsiders reported that they could see me using my hands a little more. I also resented it when my husband wanted to talk about his agenda items, because he was interrupting my sad saga. Doctors helped me see and hear more clearly, but physical and occupational therapists were the gentlest and most efficient helpers. They taught me to do what I thought I couldn't. Gradually, the "cripple" self-image went away, and I was able to take great delight in devising new ways to do things once automatic, now awkward (cutting meat, for instance). My strategy includes enjoyment, deliberately sought and cultivated, of the challenges of the pain way.

As to communication, again I was luckier than many pain persons. I have the requisite training and skill to know that communication is a two-way street. It may have been hard for me to speak honestly to doctors (I would have preferred to run away from them), but I gradually learned to do so. I also learned to listen to them, to trust them, and to help them. While I was fighting my private war against the Social Security Administration, I had access to all the doctors' reports about my hands, and the reports contained a lot of what I thought to be unnecessary information about my state of mind. A shock for anyone, and something I don't recommend to all pain persons. My initial reaction, on reading that material, was one of anger and mistrust: just like doctors to pry around in my private life! But when I read more carefully, I realized that they were only doing what had to be done, if they were to help me. I was described as "anxious," for instance, and for some reason that word made me furious. But "anxious" I was. And I would now *not* trust a doctor who wasn't able to spot the anxiety. I can even ask for observations not only from doctors, but from other outsiders.

The development of personal goals cost much in terms of time, thought, and energy. I made some very silly starts, working up ridiculous job fantasies and reading inapplicable want ads. (I at least had sense enough not to plan on being a sardine packer.) But my personal goals have begun to take shape now, and I work on them again and again. I do not assume them to be permanent, because I know better than to stake my life on anything as changeable as the pain way. I know that my primary goal is to keep on moving. I want to keep on learning.

Somewhere along the way I *did* realize that the whole issue of my pain life depended on me. Nobody else but me. I think I had already come to that realization when I dropped the onion soup. That incident helped me to take charge of myself, to understand what I could and could not do. One of the priceless psychic side-effects of "being in charge" is a genuine, highly useful sense of independence. I still make onion soup, but someone else has to lift the pot. Yet it's up to me whether it's my onion soup or Campbell's tomato.

So much for one person's development of strategy. Notice that only toward the end of the development process was I at all aware of what was going on. A great waste. Had I known how to proceed, had I realized what the pain way is like, had there been road maps for me to follow . . . but those are "if only's" and belong in the waste basket. Other pain persons will and do develop different strategies. The only advantage of an example like mine is that examples can be used as patterns against which to measure. Perhaps someone else went through what I did, although I doubt it, if for no other reason than that my hand problem is a very freaky thing. But I suspect that all pain persons travel roughly the same route. They draw up their plans. Then they—and we —can take a look at tactics, the daily maneuvers we can and do engage in.

> Strategy forms the plan of the War, and to this end it links together the series of acts which are to lead to the final decision, that is to say, it makes the plans for the separate campaigns and regulates the combats to be fought in each. As these are all things which to a great extent can only be conjectures, some of which turn out to be incorrect, while a number of other arrangements pertaining to details cannot be made at all beforehand, it follows, as a matter of course, that Strategy must go with the Army to the field in order to arrange particulars on the spot, and to make the modifications in the general plan which incessantly become necessary in War. Strategy can therefore never take its hand from the work for a moment.
>
> —*von Clausewitz*

5

Tactics, or What Works and What Doesn't

The development of a personal strategy for dealing with pain does not, of course, automatically take away the pain. Nevertheless, by coming to terms with the existence, the power, and the constancy of the intruder's threat, by treating the battle seriously, by undergoing the difficult self-assessment demanded in the creation of a strategy, the pain person can begin to make better use of available resources, both inner and outer. These resources—tactics—are the very things the pain person would like to rush to at the moment pain strikes, the quick "solutions" that look so appealing to the neophyte in pain, the "painkillers" that frequently work out so badly in actual practice. As opposed to strategy, they are functional. That is, they correspond to weaponry in war, or to the battlefield disposition of troops. The resources cover a broad range of possibilities, from meditation to distraction, from aspirin to lobotomy.

In the life of pain, all sufferers test out various tactics from time to time, although rarely do they understand that what they are doing *is* testing. Lacking that understanding, they continually undergo deep disappointment. ("That operation didn't do a damn thing for me." "Those new pills aren't any better than the other ones." "Well, honey and vinegar may work for some people, but my arthritis is still killing me.")

Tactical measures are of two kinds: personal and medical. I include in the personal category outsiders, families, and friends, and the kinds of help they offer; and in the medical category the wide spectrum of professional help. Both sets of tactics have their built-in limitations, as is true of weapons and maneuvers on the military scene. According to what I read in the papers, for instance, the Pentagon finds that the B-52 bomber, which was once the ideal airplane, has its limitations, so that we are now being invited to consider a new, improved model. I also understand that battleships have lost their place, in the national defense scheme of things, to nuclear submarines. Tactics relating to the pain way are subject to similar waves of popularity. Some kinds of surgery, once in vogue, proved not to give lasting benefits and fell from favor. So it happens that a magazine may report a new tactic and thus excite the world of pain; unhappily, we rarely read, a year or two later, a report on the disappointing performance of the same tactic.

Personal tactics sometimes take peculiar directions, directions which no pain person in search of help ought to follow. For example, pain persons, wittingly or unwittingly, often like to play games with their doctors. Richard Sternbach has devised a fascinating list of such games, a list he drew up from wide experience with the treatment of persistent pain.* Whatever their reasons, some people find great satisfaction

---

Pain Patients: Traits and Treatments (New York; Academic Press, Inc., 1974), Chapter 7.

in "getting" the doctor. Perhaps some of them anticipate making medical history with an exotic condition never before noticed by the medical profession. Perhaps some of them simply like to confuse experts, whatever the field may be. In some pain persons, there are buried feelings about doctors which surface as elements in a contest. "Getting" the doctor automatically includes such behavior as coyness and actual dishonesty even though attempts to confuse or frustrate the professional helpers generally make any help impossible. Something else is clearly going on in the heads of such pain persons—anger at the medical profession for some unexamined cause, perhaps, or an insatiable greed for more and more attention and sympathy. I do not mean to imply that such persons don't have pain; they probably do. Still, playing games, frustrating or blocking those who want to help, has very little to do with the treatment of pain, and nothing whatsoever to do with living in the pain way of life.

From the standpoint of those who must live among and with pain persons, another ill-advised choice of tactics resembles game-playing but is indulged in with other sufferers, rather than doctors. We can observe this maneuver in progress in hospitals. It can be called the "I'm sicker than you are" ploy: "My pain is worse than anyone else's." The psychological benefits derived from achieving the highest level of pain on the ward may seem somewhat offbeat to most of us, but benefits do exist, and both stoics and whimperers may play. The stiffer the upper lip, the worse the pain must be when the lip is observed to quiver; the quiet whimper that suddenly and dramatically ceases is evidence of sudden and dramatic onslaughts of severe pain. The winner is usually the pain person who makes up the rules of the game (whether it is better to be a stoic or a whimperer, whether the stoic's collapse scores higher than the whimperer's silence), thus unfailingly becoming King of the Mountain.

In this game, pain persons who can't prove that their situation is worse than everyone else's find themselves apologizing about their own trifling ailments. Ironically, these are the real winners. "He has so much more pain than I do. Am I ever lucky!" Such an attitude has positive value in the pain way. A mild form of the same supremacy struggle takes place in other settings. I am reminded of a bridge game during which every woman at the table seemed to be vying for the "Stoic of the Week" award. One was just getting over her gall bladder; another had undergone root canal work on one of her molars; the third had lower back pain and I had my hand. It made for some odd conversation during the bidding, and after a while I dropped out—not out of the bridge game, but the pain game. As I recall, the root canal lady won.

If personal tactics are sometimes unsatisfactory because there are no real battles and maneuvers going on, only counterfeit ones like the transactions in a game of Monopoly, medical tactics also sometimes leave much to be desired. Doctors also play games; a few of them play God. They have been known to play tricks on their patients in what would appear to be attempts at proving that the pain isn't as bad as reports indicated. The use and abuse of "placebos," those pills containing no medication at all that are presented as potent drugs, can serve as an example. Placebos have their place in the tactical scheme of things (sometimes they work just as well as does morphine). But the doctor who uses them to "get" the pain person, especially one who has been labeled a "crock," is playing an unattractive game.

Again, doctors have a way of calling in psychiatrists for last minute help with difficult cases of persistent pain. Why wait so long? In truth, many medical doctors and surgeons trust psychiatrists no more than do many lay people. The difficulty here is that the introduction of the psychiatrist as a last resort may make matters worse for the pain person. The intruder is hammering away at the fortress of personal integrity and suddenly the "shrink" appears. "You mean I'm *crazy?*" Whoever called in the psychiatric consultant should not have done so as a way of ridding himself or herself of an uncomfortable pain person—I mean, uncomfortable to the doctor, not the person.

Also, doctors sometimes form the bad habit of concentrating on the pain instead of the patient. Hence the temptation to refer to the "hernia in Room 415" or the "heart in Room 354." They know this problem very well, and they know how easy it is to forget that the hernia and the heart belong to human beings who do not exist in a vacuum. But sometimes they succumb to the temptation, or fail to perceive the habit. Furthermore, since the problem of pain has received increasing attention in the past ten years or so, doctors may sometimes get carried away, inadvertantly, with the impulse toward research and problem solving, so that pain persons become statistical items. Doctors, like university professors, like to publish articles. It sometimes happens that the individual sufferer turns up as a letter from the alphabet in a study of pain (Mr. A).

Given the widespread publicity surrounding the incidence of "unnecessary" surgery, it scarcely needs to be said that some surgeons love to operate. But it does need to be said that some patients love to be operated on. This, too, is a game or contest.* What is tragic about unnecessary surgery is that, for the pain person, this kind of contest is one in which he or she has the most to lose. Acute pain, caused by an operable

---

*It is interesting to note that the word "agony" comes from the Greek word for "contest" or "conflict." The Greeks used the same word for "games," as in "Olympic Games."

lesion, may well develop into persistent pain that is not treatable, or shouldn't be treated, surgically. Someday, some surgeon is going to say, "No more." And the game is over. What happens with an overabundance of surgical procedures for pain is that the pain person has been detoured. Beating a way back to the main way of pain is all the more difficult. Most pain people are less interested in conducting contests with doctors than they are with finding relief, just as most doctors are more interested in helping pain people than in joining in the game. Yet it is critically important to be aware of the peculiar things that go on, both personally and medically, within the tactical area of the pain experience.

Personal tactics in fighting pain ought to be approached in general terms, since the choice among tactics, like the master strategy, depends for its effectiveness upon individual circumstances. All pain persons make use of tactical weapons and maneuvers, whether they are consciously identified as such or not. Why then, do we need to examine tactics? There are two reasons: First, by knowing them to be only tactics, we can make more effective use of them as means to a strategic end; second, we can stop assuming that they play a primary role in the battle, that we can expect miracles from them. For example: Under normal circumstances, a headache calls for quick tactical action—we reach for the aspirin bottle. But if the headache persists, as the label on the aspirin bottle directs us, we visit the doctor's office. That visit may bring out some valuable information about what's going on in our lives. A problem comes to light, a strategy (perhaps a change in living habits) emerges, and while the aspirin bottle is still useful, its place in the strategic scheme is defined. We know what and how much to expect from it.

Knowledge of what tactical weapons can and cannot do

leads pain persons to use them judiciously, by intent rather than by accident. Once we know how and why to apply them, they work much better. Because of the particular nature of my hand problems, I can enhance the effects of my neurostimulators by rubbing the palms of my hands against my shoulders. I don't remember when it dawned on me that in so doing I was tactically reinforcing pain relief, but now that I am conscious of the effects, I deliberately take advantage of them, especially when barometric pressure drops rapidly. It probably looks a little odd, but it certainly works. If tried and true tactics don't always and everywhere apply (and they don't), they can still be tested for their value in individual cases. Out of some basic groups of personal tactics, then, the individual may be able to extract something suitable and practical for the fight.

Distraction is, I think, the single best weapon at the pain person's disposal. It has enormous advantages. For one thing, it works both physiologically and psychologically, thereby attacking the pain problem from both sides at once. As I have already noted, in recounting my own case, once the brain is actively engaged in something other than the perception of pain, the perception-response connection somehow breaks down.

Distraction is inexpensive and non-habit-forming; it does not require a doctor's prescription. As a means to the desired end, it is available everywhere and anywhere, depending on the pain person's needs. Many pain people overlook its splendid qualities, probably because it doesn't require a prescription and a lot of money. In much the same fashion, people with the flu often prefer expensive antibiotics, which usually don't work for flu anyway, to the common aspirin tablet, which does work. The virtues of distraction seem so commonplace that pain persons may not always take them seriously.

Another major advantage to distraction: It works well on all forms of pain, organic, psychogenic, and all points in between. In other words, whatever the source from which the intruder attacks, distraction keeps it at bay. The effectiveness of distraction is noted in medical literature, and pain specialists are familiar with its power. But as an applied analgesic tactic, it has so far escaped the serious attention of researchers, and few pain persons know the ways in which it works. I have learned how to distract myself from the pain experience by deliberately choosing to do so. If pain wakes me from sleep before I'm ready to get up and put on my electronic gear, I choose distraction: I plan my day, or work on a problem area in a lecture, or plan a dinner, including recipes. Sometimes I even fall back to sleep in the midst of all this.

Unfortunately, there are distractions that work and those that don't, according to individual circumstances. Television can be distracting. Even a soap opera can become a surrogate world, one in which the pain person forgets his or her own pain in favor of the ersatz pain played out on the screen in front of a comfortable chair. However, watching "Days of Our Lives" for months on end is a non-activity, and it may make the persistent pain worse, particularly LBP. Medical people generally frown on chronic TV-watching, since the body does need some activity, if only to keep its working parts in order. But there's another problem with excessive TV. Preoccupation with that ersatz pain may inhibit pain persons from developing other forms of tactics, even other forms of distraction. Furthermore, TV-watching is a solitary pastime. It is likely to reinforce the isolation of pain.

What other forms of distraction are available to the pain person? I could make up a list—in fact, I will—but my list is my own, limited to what I can think of. Pain persons from other backgrounds and with other interests will wish to add and subtract from it:

Hobbies: These can be of immeasurable value, providing they offer sufficient challenge. Whatever the hobby—needlework, gardening, woodworking, photography—it should demand attention, entail complete concentration. Normally, we think of hobbies as activities to occupy "spare" time. For the pain person, a hobby is something to absorb the mind. I know that model trains would have been a fine hobby for me, but I never got around to doing anything about it.

Parties: Pain persons may like to avoid social encounters, for reasons already touched upon. They are most likely to avoid them when in the grip of depression. But meeting and greeting do require attention, as does a change of setting. And while learning to do so may seem a hard job, listening to other people provides both distraction and a brief trip out of isolation. Going to parties requires self-discipline.

Pets: Cats, dogs, parakeets, and tropical fish cannot understand a human tale of woe. They demand a great deal of attention.

Politics: Personally, I think that nothing beats a campaign for distraction from personal pain, whether my candidate wins or loses. And it need not be a presidential campaign, either. School boards and city councils get elected. And legislators need to be watched over, if only by those who send letters to the editor. One pain person of my acquaintance gets so distracted in political seasons that people who meet him during those times of the year have no idea of the degree or duration of his pain.

Sports: These are not necessarily restricted to those who can actively participate. I have developed a spectator's taste for professional football. It's wonderfully distracting, because I find myself verbally quarreling with referees' calls, instructing the quarterback as to the plays he should call, and so on. If pain flares up in my hands, I take note of it, but it doesn't bother me. I know a man with lower back pain who can no longer play golf but who serves as an official at tournaments.

Work: It may go against the grain of those who are conditioned to think of a job as sacred, as an ethical imperative, to place "work" under the category of "distraction." But there's frequently no reason for a pain person not to work, and even a part-time job takes the pain person's eye off the place that hurts. Even when a job has crises connected with it, a crisis situation can do wonders, always providing that the crisis doesn't get entangled with whatever psychological factors are involved in pain perception. For instance, a pain person incapacitated by a psychosomatic lesion ought probably not to use a stress-loaded job for distraction; it might backfire. In fact, the merits and drawbacks of work should probably be thought about or talked over with an outside observer.

Writing: Many pain persons find that trying to "write it all out" is distracting. It requires detachment, for one thing, and, if it is to be something other than foolish self-indulgence, it demands careful use of the language, which in turn demands complete concentration. The obvious drawback to writing is the fact that, if too narrowly limited to one's own present experience, it may produce unwanted side-effects, such as self-pity. But pain persons needn't write solely about their pain.

Concentration is the key to distraction. When pain takes people to the depths, they usually find themselves concentrating on "pain-as-thing." Once they have moved away from that trap, they can consciously settle on some other "thing" to pay attention to, thus diminishing the intruder's power and cutting it down to a manageable size, as well as reducing their suffering. The choice of object or activity on which to concentrate depends on the pain person's interests, intelligence, past history, and present reality, although new objects and activities are fun to try out.

Some forms of persistent pain resist distraction, of course —no one tactic works for everyone. And some pain persons would prefer to keep on concentrating on their pain. But distraction is still the best medicine in the world. Although I have no facts or figures to prove it, I would be willing to assert that distraction works for a higher percentage of pain persons than does morphine. Anyway, it's cheaper.

Along with distraction goes a parallel tactic—*involvement*. Distraction takes the mind away; involvement brings it back, on an entirely different plane. Involvement could be translated as commitment to something outside the world of pain. At the tactical level, the pain person needs to move outside the confines of the life of pain, needs to get out of prison. Here again, individual tastes and histories help to shape the possibilities. For instance, one severely burned young man decided to write poetry. His occupational therapist encouraged him to do so, as a distraction. He soon discovered that, in order for his poetry to be good on its own merits, not just a personal distraction, he needed to take some courses in writing. Attending classes must, I think, increase his pain, but I am told that his poetry is getting better. He is now talking about student politics; his conversation reflects all the symptoms of involvement, and he shows great indignation at student apathy. The young man serves as a classic example of how distraction can lead to involvement. It is not beyond possibility that a hobby might develop in much the same manner. It is also noteworthy that involvement, for him, brought him back into the world again, if not the same world he had to abandon, at least a world other than that of oppression by pain. One pain person reported that "I found working as a volunteer at a hospital so involving that I looked forward to Saturdays and Sundays, when I could spend five hours running errands, directing strangers to the cafeteria, showing visitors which bank of elevators to take, and so on. I met all kinds of people, fascinating people; I made new friends. I became so involved in what I was doing that I had neither time nor space for my own concerns."

And one man with LBP coordinates the efforts of a group soliciting funds for the United Way. Out of his rather limited Social Security disability payments, he also manages to donate to the program. He is particularly interested in community services for the elderly and attends City Council meetings to speak his mind about such matters as the cost of public transportation.

Involvement in some activity outside the pain way of life does more than merely distract. It makes the pain way very nearly optional, if only for a few hours a day. This is not to say that the pain way has been eliminated, because it hasn't and may never be. Rather, it has temporarily been bypassed. As a traveler might choose not to take the interstate highway from Boston to New York, but to drive along the old Route 1 instead, to look at some different scenery, to escape the monotony of six-lane, high speed boredom, so the pain person can take a different route for a while. Sooner or later, both will have to return to the familiar road, and the pain person will have to carry his pain luggage with him, even on the optional route. But finding that there are alternatives provides the opened eyes and ears with something to see and hear.

Consider, once more, the physically handicapped. Most of

them learn, far more rapidly than do most pain persons, how to get involved in concerns other than themselves and their problems, however severe the problems may be. At our university, one energetic paraplegic recruited a group of handicapped students with the purpose of forming an association within which common problems and concerns could be shared. Thanks to the association's efforts, the university finally got around to installing ramps and proper parking facilities for wheelchairs.

What can pain persons involve themselves in? Again, the list extends as far as does anyone's imagination. There are possibilities in every community: clubs, fund raising drives, religious organizations, volunteer work of every sort, political activism, and so on. Pain persons would be welcome. They usually have not only time to devote, but the need to commit themselves. Unlike stereotypical "joiners," they have something more than social advantages or entertainment in mind.

But I sometimes wonder why pain persons so often stay in their isolation wards. The psychological reasons are obvious enough, but so is the imperative to break loose, to rejoin the human race.

Once the pain way has been consciously accepted, it includes a group of tactics that can only be called *good manners*. There is an etiquette of pain, something like social etiquette as described in newspaper columns. Good manners belong to the category of tactics because manners have to do with the trials of daily life, and nothing could be more daily than chronic pain. Broadly defined, good manners consist of the kinds of behavior that make other people comfortable. The good hostess, for example, noticing that a dinner guest has spilled a glass of wine, does whatever she can to put the guest at ease. In the pain way of life, the pain person with good manners does everything he or she can to put those on the outside at ease. And, conversely, those on the outside who have good manners can do a great deal to put pain persons at ease. Pain etiquette works both ways.

Here are some basic rules for pain persons to follow. They are fairly obvious, and some have been referred to in other contexts. Yet they need to be restated within the framework of tactical maneuvers, because they can prove useful in coping with the detailed requirements of the pain experience.

1. *Do not recount the history of your pain experience.*

It is not only bad form to bore everyone within hearing distance with the long sad story; it is poor tactics. Most pain persons learn this rule fairly early, if only because they perceive that no one is listening. Still, there are those who fail to notice that every human being has a pain story, that they are not the only sufferers on earth. An individual pain history not only dampens conversation; it can quickly make other people feel depressed and guilty, or, in a word, uncomfortable. And, insofar as tactics are concerned, recounting the history violates the strategic principle of new setting new goals. What happened in the past needs not to be exhumed.

Incidentally, there's a bonus to be gained from not telling one's own tale of woe. A pain person who keeps buttonholing other people to describe symptoms is actually concentrating on "pain-as-thing" again. A pain person who listens to someone else's stories without interrupting displays better manners *and* gets some distraction.

2. *Find the best ways of dealing with flare-ups of pain without making a fuss.*

Flares of pain catch by surprise, which is why they are so

difficult to cope with. The more or less constant level of pain has, perhaps, been successfully managed; and then, without advance notice, the intruder hits hard. A flare of pain is not too bad when it happens in private. In public, it may create a social dilemma: "Do I scream? Excuse myself and totter, ashen-faced, from the room? Dare I try to finish the sentence I just started?" The best general rule is the one found in books about social etiquette: Do not embarrass people in the immediate vicinity. A gasp or a bitten lip can be an attention-getter, but either one can also make other people think they have blundered or have caused pain or in some fashion have been responsible for discomfort. Responses to flares of pain can be controlled. In fact, the more often they are controlled, the more easily they can be. Each suppressed response contributes a little to the store of strength needed for the next bout, as well as to a pattern of behavior that makes the next flare-up a little more bearable. In social dilemmas, the best advice is: "Hang in there until you can gracefully remove yourself." After all, nearly all pain persons have at least a little trace of the Spartan temperament. Flares of pain, at least the kind suffered by those with chronic pain, do not last forever.

3. *Direct emotions toward proper targets.*

The proper target, as has already been observed, is not the doctor (although a pain person may take a dim view of the medical profession and consider it fair game). Nor is it family, friend, or self. For help in working out the practical details of directing emotions, pain persons may wish to consult the experts. But it is very bad manners indeed to drag everyone down to one's own pain level by misdirecting one's outbursts. It is, to be sure, foolish not to expect occasions during which emotions get out of hand—they frequently do.

Perhaps the best we can all hope for is to learn from our mistakes. Yesterday's explosion might, when observed in retrospect, yield information about better, more accurate ways of identifying the proper target—the intruder.

4. *Do as much by and for yourself as is possible; and when asked for help, give directions. Do not be deceived by the COIK fallacy.*

The COIK fallacy is the "Clear Only If Known" one. "Take the first right hand turn before you come to the covered bridge." Obviously, until we reach the covered bridge, which of us knows where the first right hand turn is? Accurate directions are based on the assumption that people really don't know how to proceed, that they wouldn't ask if they did. People who deal with pain persons need to know what is expected of them; but pain persons, operating from the common misconception that "everybody knows what it feels like," sometimes fail to give clear signals. These signals cannot be received by extra-sensory perception or necessarily by intuition. By trial and error, pain persons who know what they are doing learn what is within their capabilities. It is up to them to let others know what things are impossible. When limits have been determined and directions settled, aloud and even in writing, everyone is more comfortable, the pain person because he or she no longer has to fend off unnecessary offers of assistance, and those around him or her because they no longer feel helpless to help.

5. *Figure out what is proper behavior and what is not, according to your individual circumstances.*

Details of proper behavior have to be worked out by the individual pain person, since each has a different route to travel and a different world to live in. In general, however, "proper" behavior calls for the observance of certain conventions, certain "politenesses." Not demanding the impossible, for instance; not continually demanding the secondary gains of sympathy and attention. Anyone who has gone any distance in the pain way has already discovered the perils of these secondary gains, of course; but sometimes we all slip back into bad habits. The well-mannered pain person avoids whining and the sad, brave smile. He or she accepts as quietly as possible that the outside world was not designed for pain persons (unless, of course, there is a campaign going on to improve some small aspect of that world, in which case involvement is appropriate).

How politely pain people behave depends almost entirely on how aware they are of the pain process, how it works and how it affects them. Depression and isolation greatly diminish their capacity to think about the feelings of other people. But with insight comes an increase in sensitivity about "proper" behavior. In sum, the insightful pain person fits into the world with remarkably little commotion.

Other tips for pain people:
Take the help offered in the spirit with which it is offered. The help may be ill-advised or irritating. People on the outside are fully as ignorant about what goes on during a military battle as are those who fight it; the same state of ignorance applies to the battle of pain.

Be charitable toward those who haven't the least idea how grossly offensive are the things they say. Few people fully realize their verbal blunders for what they are. Pain persons with a sense of humor enjoy an advantage here. If a remark seems in bad taste, it is best warded off with a grin, as are most examples of human folly.

Bend the rules in favor of unbelievers, the bystanders you

117

know are discussing you. Again, ignorance about pain is more widespread than illiteracy; people with Ph.Ds may know less about the experience than does a high school drop-out and yet be more skeptical. And, of course, as skeptics sometimes turn into believers despite their unbelief, so bystanders sometimes have to learn themselves, first hand, what persistent pain is really like.

Perhaps the most important rule of all for pain persons is this: Forget what other people are doing. Enjoy your own life, and don't expect other people to enjoy it for you.

Now the rules of etiquette for non-pain persons. These rules reverse the standards. We look at the pain person as a guest. How does the well-mannered outsider behave? Under ordinary rules of etiquette, few of us have trouble picking up the information necessary to stage a wedding or a dinner party, because it's all in a book somewhere. And none of us needs much instruction in how to put guests at ease, because we do the inviting, we know who's coming to dinner, and we know what they like and dislike. Pain persons, however, fall into the general class of "unwanted" or "unknown" guests. ("Unwanted" probably because persistent pain in anyone reminds us all of our own frailness and mortality; and who really wants an intruder at a party?) Wanted or unwanted, pain persons are wished on—or intrude into—the lives of those who have no rule book to follow, no knowledge of the special circumstances of pain, and not the foggiest idea as to what arrangements must be made to put these guests at ease. How do we treat them?

1. *Those who endure persistent pain are persons, not pains, although to listen to some of them might lead us to think otherwise.*

118

This is a hard maxim to remember, particularly when the pain and the pain person hang on for years, rather than for hours. The same good rule remains in force, that is, making things as comfortable as possible, even for pain persons who break the rules of pain etiquette. Most of the time, bad-mannered pain people are unaware that there are rules.

Those who suffer the sufferers might take comfort from their own good fortune. Like a host with a large bank account and a staff of servants, non-pain people have a lot going for them. Their guests may have very little. A curious parallel between the relationship of non-pain persons to pain persons and that of the privileged and the underprivileged goes some way toward an explanation of the common tendency to treat pain persons as pains. The affluent citizen who refers to "those bums on welfare" or "those chiselers on unemployment" is engaging in what sociologists call "objectifying." That is, he is treating people as if they were things. Something of the same sort goes on when bad-mannered outsiders talk about pain people. Behind the epithet forced on a welfare recipient is a human being, whether likeable or not; behind the label pinned on a pain person is a personality under siege, and the battle has left behind some unsightly scars.

So name-calling is out. So is gossip, which, in this arena as in others, relies for its effectiveness on lack of information. What would give average pain persons a treat would be the sense that outsiders were willing to see them as something other than an emotional or social or medical disaster area.

2. *Pain persons say that they have special needs; sometimes these spoken needs must be catered to, and sometimes they must be gently overlooked.*

Once again, a delicate area, one which demands sensitivity and perception from the non-pain person. Usually it is not helpful at all to swarm over a pain person with unsolicited efforts to soothe or comfort, even when one thinks one ought to do so. Such efforts might undermine whatever feeble attempts the pain person may be making to break out of the state of siege. Furthermore, if the pain person is working out a strategy, premature and unplanned relief expeditions might wreck everything. Furthermore, even if no strategy-planning is going on, even if the pain person demands relief, sometimes it is wise to say no. Attention and sympathy, yes; but only as demonstrably needed.

Again, over-protection is bad practice. Over-protection denies the social blunderer (or pain person) the opportunity to take responsibility for a blunder. If a dinner guest spills spaghetti sauce on a treasured linen table cloth, a host or hostess will allow the guest to have the table cloth cleaned; similarly, a blundering pain person ought to be allowed to make up for occasional lapses in manners. A few hard knocks do not necessarily wound the pain person, who has grown accustomed to far worse wounds. In fact, such realistic encounters reinforce the fragile impulse toward independence and selfhood.

On the other hand, many of a pain person's needs do require special attention: bouts of depression, for instance, and fear and anxiety as they grow out of hand, and the small bruises incurred during contact with the outside world. Hard psychological knocks do need some care, if they are so punishing that the pain person is felled by them. The impulse toward independence, like a sprouting seed, needs nurture, not forcing.

3. *Give every aid and comfort to those pain persons who are trying to fight the good fight; encourage those who don't know that they can fight.*

It is relatively easy to figure out who's fighting and who isn't. Non-pain persons usually intuitively admire the fighters (although this is not always the case), intuitively frown on non-fighters. The pain way is not an easy one, for any human being, no matter what kinds of responses it elicits. To a stoic outsider, it may seem that a whimperer is a hopeless coward. In actuality, perhaps all the whimperer needs is to have his or her fighting instinct coaxed (*not* bullied) back into use. On the other hand, to an over-concerned outsider it may seem that a shell-encrusted grouch needs to be left alone, when in reality some direct action is called for if he or she is ever to break through.

One good bit of etiquette for outsiders to observe is telling the truth: telling the truth in love. Observations made by outsiders can be of enormous benefit to those in pain, but only if the observations are made without prejudice and have been laundered so as to be free from misconceptions. Any observation that encourages the pain person to examine his or her situation is good; anything that encourages blind surrender is bad.

Outsiders can do much to encourage those who are fighting. Praise and attention, of course, stiffen the determination not to surrender. But one area within which encouragement frequently is not bestowed as often or as much as it should be is the area occupied by those who seemingly have won their battles. I say "seemingly" because, as we have already seen, there are no final victories. The pain person who appears to be independent, in charge, and well-adjusted to the life of pain also needs to be noticed. All of us have short memories about disasters. We also have short memories about the experiences of pain we have observed, especially when the behavior of a pain person no longer consists principally of whining or weeping or depression. It is important to remember that the pain way is fully as lonely for the successful as for the not-so-successful.

4. Be patient. And remember that "patient" means "sufferer."
It helps the non-pain person, blessed (or cursed) with the care of a pain person, to remember whatever he or she can about physical and psychological pain. Whatever can be recaptured from one's own memory proves useful, providing always that it is not used as a shining example. Since no two pain experiences are exactly alike, we cannot expect exact correspondences in response. Perhaps I had a horrible experience of pain when I was ten years old, and I didn't cry at all, and the doctor said I was a good little patient, and everybody praised me, and I've never had an ache or a pain since that time. Fine. But the pain person with whom I must deal had a different history, and it would be rude indeed if I expected him to be just like me.

Patience never attracts much attention as a virtue, probably because the word has a passive quality about it—sitting still under a host of abuses and insults, or waiting without complaining. Since it actually means "suffering," however, outsiders might try to be patient in a different sense. Endurance perhaps is more marked by stubborn refusal to give in than by anything as unfruitful as sitting still, and endurance makes up most of the activity of being patient. We "endure" the sufferer, as the sufferer "endures" being patient; we "endure" the sufferer, as the sufferer "endures" pain. Rules for making pain persons comfortable all call for staying power, as do rules for suffering decently and in order.

So much for personal tactics. What about medical tactics? Medical tactics for dealing with persistent pain have emerged from a long history of theoretical hypotheses about pain. The history of neuroanatomy and neurophysiology, for example, has produced a goodly number of theories and an equally goodly number of tactical measures. But long before there was any such thing as neuroanatomy or neurophysiology, there were attempts to formulate theories, many of which produced the tactical and pragmatic solutions that come under the heading of folk medicine. Other kinds of theories derive from cultural and philosophical speculations about the nature of the universe. The psychic pain of depression, for instance, was, in Renaissance England, attributed to an excess of "black bile" in the system, an excess linked perhaps to astrological influences or to an imbalance in natural forces; depression was then known as "melancholia." Tactical redresses involved potions to restore the balance of fluids in the body.

With the development of anatomy as a science, and with the discovery of the activities of the nervous system, other theories were proposed and acted upon. But at about the same time that anatomy became respectable, so did the problem of the relationship between "body" and "mind," a problem that still plagues those who try to treat persistent pain. The word "psychosomatic," for example, contains both "psyche" and "body" and thus testifies to the continuing existence of the 18th century philosophical view of pain: it's either in the mind or the body or both. Contemporary re-

123

search takes another view. There seems no particular reason to analyze the development of theories about pain that have emerged during the past couple of centuries. A glance at a few will illustrate the difficulties inherent in moving from theory to tactics.

The "specificity" theory developed from the observation that there is more than one kind of nerve fiber in a given nerve. The fibers seem to specialize in carrying signals— some transmit sensation, some pain—to the spinal cord and thence to the brain, where there are centers ready to receive and code the information. In other words, nerve endings or receptors have assigned roles in the nervous system. The merit of the specificity theory is that it does account for differences among nerve fibers (some are larger than others, for instance) and does allow for the brain's predominance in the pain experience. However, it does not account for some very distressing kinds of pain, such as "phantom limb" pain, in which the patient feels pain in a non-existent arm or leg via a non-existent nerve. Nor does it account for the fact that surgical procedures designed to interrupt the transmission of pain signals have not proved very successful.

The "pattern" theory proposes central points or a central area, either in the spinal tract or in the brain, wherein nerve activity induced by a painful stimulus gets excited, and, by a sort of self-perpetuating mechanism, continues to be perceived as pain, even when the painful stimulus has stopped and when an entirely different stimulus is applied. This theory accounts for some difficult kinds of pain, particularly those kinds in which the most unlikely stimulus (say, a drop in barometric pressure) can bring on a flare of pain. But again, although surgical procedures ought to work, given the hypothesis, they notably fail.

The "gate control" theory proposes that there are nerve

cells in the spinal tract which function somewhat like gates at a railroad crossing. The transmission of information about a painful stimulus is accomplished electrically; volleys of electricity pass through relay cells to the brain, where, as we have seen, some complex transactions take place, among them perception of and response to pain. It has been found that a *non*-painful stimulus, producing other volleys of electricity, interferes with the usual activity of these pain-relay cells. Ordinarily, the "gates" are "open," and the volleys excited by pain stimuli are unimpeded. But a superimposed non-painful stimulus shuts the gates, even if only partially. Suppose I stub my toe. Without thinking about it, I rub or squeeze my toe, and the pain is allayed. What has happened is that rubbing or squeezing acts as a stimulus, producing its own electrical volleys, which effectively counteract those produced by the impact of my toe against a rock. I needn't have known about the gate control theory, but the gate control theory accounts for my instinctive action: I am creating a non-painful stimulus, so as to control the pain.

Similarly, by sending its own signals, the brain can also exercise some effect on the pain relay cells, since the brain generates its own electricity and since the nervous system works both ways. So the gate control theory accounts for the results achieved by such tactics as distraction. If I am concentrating on the pain in my toe, thinking and worrying about a fracture or a sprain, the gates are apparently open. If my attention is elsewhere, the gates are apparently partially shut.

This theory accounts for a wide number of observations made both by researchers and by pain persons. It even accounts for some folk medicine, such as the advice about putting your leg in cold water immediately, if you go walking barefoot in a patch of stinging nettles. Cold and heat are stimuli and start those volleys of electricity that inhibit the painful ones. The gate control theory has been confirmed by clinical findings, both in animals and in human beings. And it has far-reaching tactical consequences.

What tactics have emerged from all the theories, whether ancient or modern?

The most obvious tactic is one that has been in use since recorded time, long before the proliferation of medical knowledge that we have today. Although ancient civilizations may not have known much neurophysiology, they knew what worked, and they very early learned one medical tactic: Do something to the brain, where the perception-response transaction is taking place.* The Greeks knew about the multi-talented opium seed, for example. Aspirin, or at least the virtues of chewing on twigs of a willow or poplar tree, is a lot older than the German chemist who learned how to synthesize its excellent properties. The Romans and the Chinese both knew about henbane, a plant whose seeds contain chemicals now used to make scopolamine, a drug used to render a surgical patient unconscious before the anesthesiologist gets to work. Wine was known to have certain advantages, and I guess it still does. The tradition of using drugs that act to numb or addle the brain has a long, and honorable, history.

There are two kinds of drugs normally used to control pain. One group is called "narcotic," the other "hypnotic." Within the past few years, a third group—the anti-seizure drugs—have been added to the pharmacological arsenal, and

---

*Guido Majno has written a stunningly thorough account of medical and surgical treatments used in ancient civilizations. *The Healing Hand: Man and the Wound in the Ancient World* (Cambridge: Harvard University Press, 1975).

drugs that control heart irritability seem also to have an effect on pain.

Both narcotic and hypnotic drugs work on the general nervous system, but they have different effects. Obviously, "narcotic" drugs have to do with "sleep." Narcotic drugs—and they come under many different trade labels—are designed to put the brain to sleep. Morphine is one. It does indeed put the brain to bed, as anyone who has ever taken it will agree: no pain—but then, no brain. Demerol is another narcotic. Codeine is another. As everyone knows by now, narcotics are addictive, and, in consequence, physicians are reluctant to prescribe them, except in limited amounts and for severe pain. However, the inevitability of addiction, as well as the concept of narcotics as addictive, has been challenged.* And there is evidence that when narcotics are administered for pain, any addictive after-effects are short-lived. Apparently, putting the brain to bed does have its attractions; but most pain persons prefer to be awake.

If narcotics work on the brain as a receiver of information, hypnotics work on the brain as perceiver. Hypnotic drugs, and some surgical procedures which accomplish much the same sort of effect, alter our perception of what's going on, both in the body and outside it. Common names for hypnotics are familiar: marijuana, LSD, peyote, and so forth. Hypnotic drugs are usually frowned upon by various segments of society, primarily because once perception of pain is altered, perception of other human experiences is also altered. Alcohol, for instance, is probably the most common of all hypnotic drugs. It induces what I have already referred to as the "I don't care" frame of mind. (This leads me to wonder if

---

*Thomas B. Hackett, "Surgical Intervention To Relieve Pain," in *Pain: Clinical and Experimental Perspectives,* ed. Matisyohu Weisenberg (St. Louis: The C. V. Mosby Company, 1975), p. 278.

marijuana works as a painkiller. I never tried it, so I cannot testify.) Hypnotics, like narcotics, have their place in the pain way. But they also have their dangers and drawbacks.

Drugs are mysterious substances, by and large. Why do not all pain people get relief from this one or that? Why do some drugs work and some not? How common is addiction? In the case of patients with advanced cancer, nobody worries about addiction, because the patient will be dead long before the problem upsets anyone. But what about the patient who isn't going to die? Placebos, when administered under what is called a "double blind" situation (that is, nobody—doctor, nurse, or patient—knows what's in the pill), work as well as morphine. Why drugs, including placebos, affect us as they do, is not yet clear.

Yet the oddities uncovered by research in pharmacology suggest once again that the individuality of the pain experience has a decided effect on the usefulness of a particular drug. Perhaps the individual's own body chemistry, which would automatically include a great many variables, also affects the results. Most assuredly, one's own history of pain does. Normally, we expect drugs to dull pain. If, on several occasions in the past, acute pain has proved beyond the reach of aspirin, we may find aspirin ineffective against persistent pain, a not altogether unpredictable reaction, given our bondage to the vocabulary of acute pain and our commitment to the notion that pain is pain, whatever its size or shape. Actually, aspirin is one of the best and safest drugs around.

In any event, whatever the prescribed drug, there is no guarantee that it will work 100% of the time for 100% of pain persons. Drugs have their uses, but their uses are limited. No magic is to be found in the drugstore.

The use of *biofeedback* as a means for control of pain

response enables the sufferer to manage his own experience to a remarkable degree. Its good effects depend on slow and carefully monitored training. The electrical signals produced by muscle tissue are amplified and thus measured. When the pain person is trained in deep relaxation, he or she can control what were once thought to be involuntary muscular responses to pain. Biofeedback seems especially effective in the treatment of migraine headaches and the muscular spasms frequently associated with lower back pain. As is the case with behavior modification, once the sequence of stimulus-perception-response is interrupted, the pain experience is altered; the pain person is once again in charge. However, even strong advocates of biofeedback warn that not all forms of the pain experience—and not all pain people—benefit from the treatment. It is not clear whether it would have much to offer someone undergoing, say, phantom limb pain or pain resulting from nerve damage.

Still on the far horizon is the prospect of tactical use of *chemical substances* found in the brain and nervous system during an attack of pain. It is common clinical knowledge that the transmission and storage of pain information depends on what might be called a "favorable" chemical climate. Morphine, for instance, alters that climate. It would seem logical, then, for biochemical research to seek a chemical alteration in the pain transaction, one that would do what morphine does, without the ugly side-effects. The prospect is indeed alluring. Yet the nervous system has a well-documented tendency to adjust itself to tactical maneuvers; when a nerve is severed, for instance, other nerves take over its work. The alteration of chemical substances may be an answer, but pain people must, as always, be patient. In any event, it will be a long time before the data now being collected can result in help for the average person.

129

Another set of medical tactics belongs to the world of surgery. Here, too, reports of results are mixed; and once more the specific tactics employed by neurosurgeons depend on theory, depend on whether they see the problem as located in the brain or in some part of the pathway followed by the transmitting mechanisms. There are two common groups of surgical tactics: Operate on the brain, the receptor; or operate on the nerve or nerves doing the transmitting. Most surgical procedures have drawbacks, as is true of any surgery for anything. There *are* risks. But most pain persons who ask for surgical relief know little about what they are demanding. Even when told about the risks, they seem not to hear. In the surgical level of tactics, then, communication between doctor and patient is of utmost importance.

Operations on the brain for relief of pain are supposed to stop pain in its tracks by excising or severing the physiological pathways in the pain process or by excising the pathways leading to the memory bank or severing connections within the memory bank. Operations on the nerve or nerves or on the transmitting junctions are supposed to stop pain by interrupting the path before the volleys can reach the brain. Unfortunately, there are many cases in which patients who have undergone multiple surgical treatments for persistent pain have had no relief whatsoever. In some cases, these patients have been suffering from psychogenic pain which, although its origin may have been organic, has retained dominance over their lives. In other cases, no surgical relief was possible, because of the nature of the lesion. More ominously, sometimes other nerves, as if trying to repair the damage done by the surgeon, take up the work of the excised nerve. And nerves can regenerate themselves. For whatever the reason, surgical relief is not always effective. Like drugs, the scalpel works on individuals, not on pain.

A relatively new surgical form of relief does not involve much cutting at all, or else none. This is neurostimulation, the kind of relief I got. Neurostimulation is based on the gate control theory. It replaces the pain sensation with something else, by providing a second stimulus, which counteracts that which produces pain. Neurostimulators activate some nerve fibers to the detriment of other sensory fibers in place of pain fibers. Some stimulators are implanted, some are affixed to the skin above the offending nerve. What results is a buzzing sensation tnat somehow overrides pain. True, there are wires to be coped with and transmitters to be carried about the body. But any surgery involved is reversible, unlike brain surgery. An implant can be removed, but an excised nerve or portion of the brain cannot be replaced. Yet one pain person I have heard of sampled neurostimulation and couldn't stand the buzzing sensation. I guess she preferred pain.

Then there's hypnosis, and I tried it and found it good, if for a brief period only.* Hypnosis, known once upon a time as "mesmerism," after the name of the man who popularized it, is not a tactic applicable to every pain person. Some are not good subjects. Essentially, hypnosis works in much the same manner as does distraction, although it is far more carefully structured and administered. The subject focuses his or her attention on something external to the body: the voice of the hypnotherapist, plus an object on which to fix the eye. Concentration of eye and ear allows the patient's imagination to take charge, under the therapist's direction, and, step by step, images replace whatever in the waking

---

*"Hypnosis" and "hypnotic" drugs are somehow connected, if only because they wear similar name tags.

state is hurting the pain person. It might be pointed out that hypnotism is not something to be practiced by amateurs. For pain persons, the best hypnotherapists are M.D.s who are trained in the art. (My hypnotherapist happens to be a childs' psychiatrist.) As the waking state recedes, so does pain. It is perceived distantly, as if the intruder were at work on someone else. Most commonly, hypnosis produces the same effects as do some drugs: "I know that there is pain going on, but it doesn't bother me." When surgeons perform lobotomies, the same effect occurs. Pain is acknowledged but does not bother.

One asset of hypnotherapy is that it taps the individual's own inner resources of imagination, rather than the spinal column; it allows for one's personal history and can apply to more than one kind of pain. So far as I know, it does no damage. To a pain person in acute distress, it is a blessing, since any relief from pain brings a sense of refreshment, a chance to rebuild and recover hope, both sorely needed. The problem, of course, is where does the pain person find a well trained hypnotherapist? And suppose he or she turns out not to be a good subject? Self-hypnosis can be taught, to be sure; but in everyday life it is not always possible to put together the necessary ingredients of inner quiet and concentration to use it when necessary. (Yet I can still hypnotize myself, given the right circumstances, back into an imagined room with a comfortable chair, my favorite music playing, and a white kid glove on my right hand. And I can still hear the sound of Dr. H's voice.)

Acupuncture is big business in the field of pain tactics, and medical literature now waxes fat with articles on how and why it works. Some observers are convinced that acupuncture, like hypnosis, depends for its effectiveness on the "suggestibility" of the subject. That is, the patient, convinced that twirling needles deaden pain, has no pain, because he or she know that needletwirling kills pain.

There are two theories about pain underlying the use of acupuncture. One of them, the ancient Chinese one, is elaborately intertwined with a Far Eastern understanding of anatomy that is metaphysical in nature. There are "forces" within the body that can be put to use in various combinations and localities so as to achieve the correct balance for combating pain. The other theory matches that of gate control. And from whatever theoretical basis one looks at acupuncture, one can notice strong psychological factors. A group of Canadian doctors observed that the Chinese have few facilities for general anesthesia, particularly in rural areas; they also observed that Chinese patients *know* that acupuncture works, both for surgical procedures and for or surgical procedures and for persistent pain.*

One doctor trained in acupuncture tells me that one of the pressing problems in the acceptance of acupuncture in pain relief is that there are a lot of quack practitioners abroad in the land. She says that acupuncture works well with certain patients, not well with others. It does not work for patients with psychogenic pain. It does work for lower back pain, because the needles can stimulate the muscles to the point of exhaustion, whereupon they relax and cease hurting.

More research into the cause-effect theory of acupuncture has to be done—on this, everyone agrees. In the meantime, patients going to an acupuncturist should be sure that the

---

*Leonard C. Jenkins and Wolfgang E. Spoered, "Acupuncture: Canadian Anesthetist Report on a Visit to China," *Canadian Medical Association Journal,* Vol. III, No. 10: p. 1123.

person handling the needles is an M.D., that a proper diagnosis has been made, that acupuncture is an appropriate tactic. Copper bracelets for the relief of arthritic pain are relatively harmless. Acupuncture may be dangerous unless carried out by a competent physician who has made a thorough physical examination.

The biggest tactical news in recent years has been the development of what are known as *pain clinics.* The pain clinic is designed to treat the whole person, including his or her own personal history, family history of pain, personality, and all the other small circles included in the diagram in Part III. A pain clinic is staffed not only by medical doctors and nurses, but by psychiatrists, psychologists, physical and occupational therapists, and social workers. Assuming that the primary lesion or disease has been taken care of, treatment centers on the patient's *response* to persistent pain. If he or she needs detoxification (many pain persons do, after years of drugs), this is done. But addiction to those familiar secondary gains also needs attention. Those gains (sympathy, coddling, and the like) are withdrawn; the patient is given attention when he or she does not complain, is treated with detached neutrality when he or she does. By waiting an extra hour for a pain pill, for instance, the pain person receives a different set of secondary gains: "Great! That's wonderful!" replaces "Oh, you poor, poor thing!" The retraining of the response end of the pain experience is found to alter the perception of it.

Obviously, the pain clinic tactics develop from an understanding of pain as something more than a physical sensation; their tactics rely heavily on the psychological and social components of the experience. They report a high rate of success; but they also report some failures. The reported failures seem to be among those whose pain is more precious than any cure. The psychological premise upon which they depend is that of "behavior modification," popularized by B. F. Skinner. If a pain person resists that premise, of course, a pain clinic will probably not work out well. The great advantage of clinic procedures is the stated objective of treating the whole person.

Physical and occupational therapy together constitute one of the best and one of the least appreciated tactical endeavors available to pain persons. It is a pity that more physicians do not understand the value of these forms of therapy.

Physical therapy helps the pain person to regain and retain the use of muscles and joints that may have, in a domino-effect, become affected by persistent pain. In their fright and anxiety, pain persons literally get uptight. By treating those muscles and joints—whirlpool baths, passive and active exercise, and so forth—the physical therapist coaxes forth as much activity as possible. And when a painful joint or muscle is a little more active, there is a little less pain.

Occupational therapy has nothing to do with vocational counseling. It is a mode of treatment designed to produce maximum use of the parts of the body that have been damaged by persistent pain—like my hands. It teaches skills, sometimes skills that a toddler has but that an adult has lost. Occupational therapy enabled me to regain a great deal: I was taught how to cut a piece of meat, how to manage my wayward fingers and thumbs in picking up objects, how to open doors.

The two branches of therapy work together and achieve truly remarkable results. But they have their limitations. Some pain persons simply lack the motivation necessary to see physical and occupational programs through. Others are not prime candidates, because of the nature of their lesions. Yet physical and occupational therapy, like many other tactics, does no harm. And, I might add, among all those who helped me along my way, the physical and occupational therapists were the most pleasant and cheerful.

The important thing to notice about medical tactics is that no single one can guarantee total success. Drugs, surgery, hypnosis, pain clinics, physical and occupational therapy, all have limitations. The pain way of life is so complex that no single remedy will work for everyone. It is so complex, in fact, that without a strategy, the common practice of running from one tactical experiment to another turns out to be dispiriting, exhausting, and depressing.

In general, when picking and choosing among tactical offerings, it seems best that the pain person have some idea why he or she thinks something will work. If acupuncture doesn't work, forget it; but keep in mind that it didn't work. But why acupuncture in the first place? A personal strategy might include sampling a number of different possibilities; but if that is the case, the master plan has to include the possibility of failure along with the others.

The gravest error of all is to limit strategy to a single tactical measure. That way lies only grief, discouragement, and surrender.

> Tactics and strategy are two activities mutually permeating each other in time and space, at the same time essentially different activities, the laws and mutual relations of which cannot be intelligible at all to the mind until a clear conception of the nature of each activity is established.
>
> —*von Clausewitz*

Epilogue

In the strictest sense, there can be no epilogue to the pursuit of pain, since "epilogue" means "concluding statement, a summary or a speech given by an actor after the play is over." Pain and its pursuit keep going, and pain is neither a speech, a literary work, nor a play. But a prologue implies an epilogue, and, in any case, we still have to do something about Mr. A, who, with a large group of fellow-sufferers, was in poor condition when last seen. We, outsiders and insiders alike, can sometimes afford a resting point in the pursuit; so we can stop a moment and try to find a way to get him on his feet. At least it is time to say something about what might have been, what might still be, not only for him, and his wife and family and friends, but for all pain persons and their helpers who are stranded, alone, frightened, angry, and depressed.

In an ideal world, one made up of ideal pain persons, doctors, families, friends, and institutions, Mr. A would have found himself surrounded by people who completely com-

137

prehended the pain process. He himself would have understood it. He would have *known,* for instance, that the pain might recur; he would have had psychiatric help from the beginning, and his wife and family would have had counseling. He would have comprehended the nature of the intruder, and so would those having to treat him or live with him. And, since he would have been an ideal pain person, he would never have chosen to live in a shell. He would have embarked on the pain way of life with his eyes open. In that ideal world, Mr. A would have constructed his new "home" with care; he would have settled on the tactics appropriate to his way; he would be, if not free of the intruder, at least as whole a personality as anyone on the outside.

But when we conjured up Mr. A, we didn't put him in an ideal world. We placed him in the world as it is. Nobody educated him. Nobody told him all that persistent pain might do to him. As it happened, he did not get the help he needed when he most needed it, and there he is, in his shell. Can we pry him out, now that he has signed a lease on the place? Some bystanders might say "Why bother?" Pain persons, and those who deal with them, know better, know who Mr. A is and might be.

Someone will, in all probability, have to confront him with the facts of his life, with what is going on. And whoever confronts him—his wife, his children, his family doctor, his surgeon—will surely have to undergo some heavy emotional weather, because pain persons who have decided not to fight show a remarkable capacity to fight those who wish to help. Those who do the confronting need compassion, courage, and wit, in order to let the storms ride themselves out.

Telling a chronic pain person the truth requires loving concern, and loving concern sometimes includes bluntness. If a pain person is a grouch or a whiner, that is a fact, one which may legitimately be identified. If a pain person is driving his family into a swamp of guilt feelings with that sweet, sad suffering, that too is a fact. Pain persons have to know the truth about themselves before they can begin to move forward. But facts are best communicated dispassionately and without the bitter additives of resentment and anger. Thus, whoever confronts Mr. A also needs to be detached. Assuredly, it is better for him to learn late than never; but he, like other pain persons, cannot learn what he cannot hear, and if the facts are told in such a manner that he will not listen, he will remain exactly where he is.

One of the commonplace statements made about pain in medical literature is that "it" is a complex phenomenon. Indeed "it" is, and why the word gets stressed so much ought to come as no surprise. Human beings are themselves complex, and the difficulties associated with the treatment of pain grow out of complexity. Yet within all the twists and turns that the pain way of life takes, the way remains one that most human beings have to take, at some time or other. How they manage it remains a matter of conscience as much as skill, as does the matter of how other people manage them.

One more thing. Pain persons frequently feel themselves unable to accomplish much of anything. Yet they can make an important contribution to the world at large. The more they manage to conduct themselves with dignity, to live out their lives with a modest degree of humor and insight, the more they encourage non-pain persons to face *their* own terrors, whatever those may be. Few pain persons ought to force themselves to be glowing examples of courage and bravery and fortitude, twenty-four hours a day, seven days a week. We all have our bad moments. And I don't suppose for a moment that practice ever made perfect, in the pain way. Still, since pain is probably the most dreaded threat (persons with terminal cancer are said to fear death a lot less than they do the prospect of extreme pain), pain persons can show the world how to live with it.

After all, pain is a way of life. On the whole, I think it's better than no life at all.

Bibliography

The following list of works is in no sense designed to be a complete bibliography for research in the problem of pain. In the past five years, the literature about the subject has grown in what seems a geometric progression. Many of the works cited are not available to the lay person, but some are. I have marked with an asterisk those which seem to me to be most useful in providing a general view of pain. For more specific literature, these works afford their own bibliographic references.

Basmajian, John V. "Pain Control in Physical Rehabilitation." (tape recording) Biomonitoring Applications, Inc., New York, 1976.
Bond, M. R. "The Relation of Pain to the Eysenck Personality Inventory, Cornell Medical Index, and Whitely Index of Hypochondriasis." *British Journal of Psychiatry,* Vol. 119, 1971, p. 617.
*Bonica, John J. and Black, R. G. "The Management of a Pain

Clinic." *Relief of Chronic Pain*, ed. Mark Swerdlo. *Excerpta Medica*. Vol. 1, 1974.

Bonica, John J.; Procacci, Paolo; and Pagni, Carlo A. *Recent Advances on Pain: Pathophysiology and Clinical Aspects*. Springfield, Ill.: Charles C. Thomas, 1973.

Bowsher, D.; Mumford, J.; Liptom, S.; and Miles, J. "Treatment of Intractable Pain by Acupuncture." *Lancet*, Vol. 2, 1973, p. 57.

Craig, Kenneth L. and Weiss, Stephen M. "Vicarious Influences on Pain Threshold Determinations." *Journal of Personal Sociology and Psychology*, Vol. 19, 1971, p. 53.

Davidson, Park O. and Neufeld, Richard W. J. "Response to Pain and Stress: A Multivariate Analysis." *Journal of Psychosomatic Research*, Vol. 18, 1974, p. 25.

*Davitz, Lois J.; Sameshima, Yasuoko; and Davitz, Joel. "Suffering as Viewed in Six Different Cultures." *American Journal of Nursing*, Vol. 76, 1976, p. 1296.

*Edelstein, E. L. "Experience and Mastery of Pain." *Israel Annals of Psychiatry and Related Disciplines*, Vol. 12, 1974, p. 216.

Elkins, Alan M. "Other Meanings of Symptoms." *Journal of the Maine Medical Association*, Vol. 64, 1973, p. 91.

Fordyce, W. E. "Operant Conditioning as a Treatment Method in Management of Selected Chronic Pain Problems." *Northwest Medicine*, Vol. 69, 1970, p. 580.

Gatz, Arthur J. *Manter's Essentials of Clinical Neuroanatomy and Neurophysiology, 4th Edition*. Philadelphia: F. A. Davis Company, 1973.

Gentry, W. Doyle; Shows, W. Derek; and Thomas, Michael. "Chronic Lower Back Pain: a Psychological Profile." *Psychosomatics*, Vol. 15, 1974, p. 174.

*Graham, David T. "Health, Disease, and the Mind-Body Problem: Linguistic Parallelism." *Psychosomatic Medicine*, Vol. 29, 1967, p. 52.

Hart, F. Dudley. *The Treatment of Chronic Pain*. Philadelphia: F. A. Davis Company, 1974.

Jenkins, Leonard C. and Spoerel, Wolfgang E. "Canadian Anesthetists Report on a Visit to China." *Canadian Medical Asso-*

ciation Journal, Vol. III, No. 10, 1974, p. 1123.

Johnson, Jean E. "Effects of Accurate Expectations About Sensations on the Sensory and Distress Components of Pain." *Journal of Personal and Social Psychology,* Vol. 27, 1973, p. 261.

Loeser, John D. "Dorsal Rhizotomy for the Relief of Chronic Pain." *Journal of Neurosurgery,* Vol. 36, 1972, p. 745.

*Majno, Guido. *The Healing Hand: Man and the Wound in the Ancient World.* Cambridge: Harvard University Press, 1975.

Mastrovito, Rene C. "Psychogenic Pain." *American Journal of Nursing,* Vol. 74, 1974, p. 514.

Mattsson, Ake. "Long-Term Physical Illness in Childhood: a Challenge to Psychosocial Adaptation." *Pediatrics,* Vol. 50, 1972, p. 601.

Mechanic, David. "Social and Psychological Factors Affecting the Presentation of Bodily Complaints." *New England Journal of Medicine,* Vol. 286, 1972, p. 1132.

*Melzack, Ronald and Torgerso, W. S. "On the Language of Pain." *Anaesthesiology,* Vol. 34, 1971, p. 50.

Melzack, R. "Phantom Limb Pain: Implications for Treatment of Pathologic Pain." *Anaesthesiology,* Vol. 34, 1971, p. 409.

*Melzack, Ronald. *The Puzzle of Pain.* New York: Basic Books, 1973.

Nashold, Blaine S., Jr. and Friedman, Harry. "Dorsal Column Stimulation for Control of Pain." *Journal of Neurosurgery,* Vol. 56, 1972, p. 590.

Ostrow, Lynne Stanton. "New Hope for Patients with Trigeminal Neuralgia." *American Journal of Nursing,* Vol. 76, 1976, p. 1301.

Pilowsky, I. and Spence, N. D. "Patterns of Illness Behaviour in Patients With Intractable Pain." *Journal of Psychosomatic Research* (Oxford), Vol. 19, 1975, p. 279.

Pos, Robert. "Psychological Assessment of Factors Affecting Pain." *Canadian Medical Association Journal,* Vol. 111, 1974, p. 1213.

Rosillo, R. H. and Fogel, M. L. "Correlation of Psychologic Variables and Progress in Physical Rehabilitation: Degree of Disability and Denial of Illness." *Archives of Physical Medicine and Rehabilitation,* Vol. 51, 1970, p. 227.

*Sternbach, Richard A. *Pain Patients: Traits and Treatment.* New York: Academic Press, 1974.

Szasz, T. S. *Pain and Pleasure: A Study of Bodily Feelings.* New York: Basic Books, 1957.

Szasz, T. S. "The Psychology of Persistent Pain." *Pain,* ed. A. Soulaire et al. London: Academic Press, 1968, p. 93.

Walters, A. "Psychogenic Regional Pain Alias Hysterical Pain." *Brain,* Vol. 84, p. 1.

Weisenburg, Matisyohu, ed. *Pain: Clinical and Experimental Perspectives.* St. Louis: The C. V. Mosby Co., 1975.

White, J. C., and Sweet, W. H. *Pain and the Neurosurgeon.* Springfield, Ill.: C. C. Thomas, 1974.

Woodforde, J. M., and Mersky, H. "Some Relationships between Subjective Measures of Pain." *Journal of Psychosomatic Research,* Vol. 16, 1972, p. 173.